THE CALIFORNIA WEIGHT CLINIC PROGRAM

How to become a
Down-Sizer!

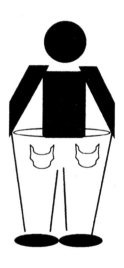

*Five Easy-to-Follow Steps to
What it Really Takes
to Control Your Weight*

Paul Stevens, Ph.D.

How to Become a Down-Sizer!
The California Weight Clinic Program
© 2002
Paul Stevens, Ph.D.

ISBN 0-9720253-0-8
Library of Congress Control Number: 2002092049

BRASS HAT PRESS

P.O. BOX 2127
SONOMA, CA 95476

Printed in the U.S.A. by
Morris Publishing
3212 East Highway 30
Kearney, NE 68847
1-800-650-7888

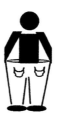

How to Become a
DOWN-SIZER!

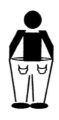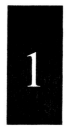

What it *Really Takes* to Control Your Weight

Congratulations! You have taken the first step on the road to taking control of your life and your weight. For many of you, this is but one more step on a long road toward weight control.

Your perseverance is testimony to your spirit and commitment. I am confident that the principles in this book can help you reach and maintain your goals.

How to Become a Down-Sizer! synthesizes the process of losing and controlling your weight into a few easy-to-follow steps that you can really use. After reading this book, you will be armed with the information you need to lose and control your weight.

The DOWN-SIZER SYSTEM does not befuddle you with excessive information or confound you with difficult to follow rules, recipes, or regulations. The methods are simple and straightforward, designed to help promote a healthy lifestyle, and will give you the tools you need to control your weight. This easy-to-follow five point plan includes changes that really work that you can begin implementing today.

Congratulations! You are on your way.

DOWN-SIZING

Anyone who has ever had excess weight to deal with probably already has a wealth of information. You have probably read all the books, been to this or that program, or used one system or another. However, what most of us are missing are just the basics about what it really takes to lose weight.

Becoming a "Down-Sizer" is not a diet, but instead, a way to live. It is simply a matter of applying some easy-to-understand principles to your life, adding a few ideas to the way you think about eating and food, and implementing a few actions in your daily life.

Let's concentrate on what it really takes to achieve and maintain a healthy weight. It's not that complicated, and it's not that hard to do.

THE ROLE OF GENETICS IN WEIGHT LOSS

Getting the Right Attitude

As we get started, I would like to point out the role and importance of genetics in weight control. Research has shown that being overweight is, in most cases, a genetic condition.

If you are overweight, you most probably have a genetic disposition to being so. There is probably a history of being overweight in your family, and you may have parents or siblings who are also overweight.

This was a good thing back in the cave days when we did not know where our next meal was coming from. Those of us who tended to hold on to extra fat were the survivors.

But we no longer live in caves. Now there is a fast food restaurant on every corner, and snack machines down in the break room. A slow metabolism and a trait to store and hold on to fat is no longer necessary. It is no longer an advantage. These days it works against us.

Of course, we get a lot of good things from our parents: our good looks, our intelligence, perhaps our sense of humor! But every so often we get a thing or two we might be better off without. The tendency to be overweight is one of these things. It is passed down in the genes, like hair color, freckles, or other physical features.

What About Psychology?

Sure, there are psychological factors to being overweight. People learn unhealthy habits. Some people eat during times of stress or when they are bored or to stuff down their emotions or to satisfy some unsatisfied need or desire.

But, even those of you who do overeat for some psychological reason probably have a genetic component to being overweight. You probably know (and perhaps secretly or not so secretly, dislike) people who can eat anything they want and not gain weight.

There are people out there who overeat, snack all night long, or eat in unhealthy ways, and yet they do not have a problem with their weight. Some people seem to eat anything they want - any time they want - and never gain a pound. Others among us can do little more than glance at a piece of chocolate and gain weight.

Why is this? It's not fair! But, there it is. What can you do?

What Can You Do?

Gee, I'm glad you asked, and I'll get to that in a minute.

In the meantime, the point of talking about genetics is to stress that if you are overweight it is not your fault. It is a condition you were born to experience.

Often people blame themselves for being overweight. And, all too often, they have been blamed by many others, including their doctors, in subtle - and sometimes not so subtle - ways.

But if you are overweight, it does not mean that you have a psychological problem or that there is something wrong with you. Yes, there may be psychological factors involved, but your weight is much more likely to be related to your genetic makeup than to your psychology.

The reason some people can eat what they want without gaining weight has to do with their metabolism, or the rate at which the body transforms food into energy. To complicate matters, as we age and grow older, our metabolism tends to slow down. So, it happens that many people who have never had a weight problem wake up one day, look in the mirror, and ask "Where did all this weight come from?"

So, the answer to "What can you do?" is simple. You need to increase your metabolism, which will in turn burn more fat. And we will be talking about just how to do that.

The past does not equal the future

You are not doomed or destined to repeat your own personal history. As you begin striving for - and achieving - a healthy weight, it is important to remember that you are not overweight because you are weak or somehow psychologically damaged. In fact, it is quite the contrary. As you begin to succeed and reach your weight goals, you will be demonstrating a great deal of strength, commitment and willpower.

Since the tendency to gain and hold on to weight is most probably part of your genetic make up, it will be with you the rest of your life. I do not say this to discourage you, but rather to point out that you will always need to pay attention to your eating and lifestyle habits, much like a person with diabetes has to pay attention to what her or she eats, or a person with allergies has to avoid certain plants or animals.

Therefore, it is important that you plan to change your habits permanently. Begin to think of yourself as a person who will exercise and eat in a healthy manner, no matter what life may bring. Don't go on a diet, but instead, start eating in a new way. The good news (and there is plenty of good news to go around) is that you do not have to change everything overnight.

It took years for you to put on your extra weight, and it will take some time to take it off. In that time you can begin to develop new habits - and a new way of looking at life - that will help you become the person you desire to be.

There may be hurdles, and even slips and falls along the way. Maybe your family resists your new lifestyle. Maybe you just can not find enough time right now. Maybe this. Maybe that. Nonetheless, keep your goal in mind. Everyday take small steps toward your goal. Everyday take aim toward developing new habits and new ideas that will serve you for the rest of your life.

And, here's even more good news...it's easier than you may think!

...GO!

THE *5* POINTS OF THE DOWN-SIZER SYSTEM

The Necessary Ingredients to Weight Control

Let's get to it.

There are five main points in learning to control your weight. These five points are:

Exercising

Eating a low-fat diet

Controlling portions

Avoiding refined sugars

Not skipping meals

With these five simple, and easy-to-follow, steps you can, and will, be able to control your weight.

Let's take them one at a time.

DOWN-SIZER
STEP #1

EXERCISE

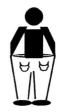

(The dreaded, and oh so misunderstood, case of...)

Some moderate exercise is probably the most important aspect of the Down-Sizer program. It is by far the best predictor of who will or will not succeed in controlling their weight. Yeah, yeah, everybody knows you're supposed to exercise. But who has the time or the money to join a gym, or the sustained inspiration, or a thousand-and-one other objections that come rushing to mind?

For me, this was always the point at which I would simply turn off the discussion in my mind.

...but wait, there is more good news on the way...

WHAT KIND OF EXERCISE?

Exercising does not mean you have to join a gym, take a Jazzersize class, jump up and down on boxes, or climb up and down on a Stairmaster until you faint. All your body needs is some moderate aerobic exercise, and for that, a brisk walk will do nicely.

Aerobic literally means "with air" or "to exercise with air." It is not necessary for you to do the aerobic type of exercise that is designed to improve and condition your heart and lungs. Of course, if you are already doing it, that is fine. But even if you can not exercise strenuously, you can still do what is needed for weight control.

"Aerobic exercise" - for our purposes - is just what it takes to work up a bit of a sweat or get your heart rate a little faster than usual.

Increasing your heart rate will in turn increase your metabolic level, which in turn increases the rate at which your body burns fat. Simple.

GO FOR A WALK

There is some debate over how long the metabolic effects of aerobic exercises last. But everyone is agreed that it is an essential part of any weight loss program.

Some studies have shown that once you get your metabolic rate up, it lasts for up to a day and a half. This means once you increase your metabolism, it will continue burning fat all the time, even when you are not exercising. You will simply have a faster - higher - metabolism. This will burn more fat. This will happen while you are exercising and will continue to occur while you are sleeping, driving your car, and doing anything else.

So, if you plan to exercise every other day (plus one) or four times per week, you will be able to keep your metabolism up at a higher rate. In order to increase and maintain your metabolic rate, try exercising for thirty minutes at a time. Aim for walking three miles in under an hour.

When we participate in sustained exercise out bodies tend to burn sugars during the first twenty minutes or so. It is after this point that we start burning fat. Even if you do not burn off that many calories, you will be reconditioning your metabolism to work at a higher rate. Your body will use your food as energy today, instead of storing it as fat.

One sure and easy way to increase your metabolic rate is to go for a walk. Walking is nice. It is something most people can do. And it does not take a lot of extra equipment, clothes, money or other special requirements.

Of course, some people cannot walk for some physical reason. And, while we are on the subject, if you haven't exercised for awhile, take it easy as you get started. Talk to your doctor if you have any questions about your health and the risks of exercising. And most importantly, don't overdo it. It will not do you any good to hurt yourself by getting excited and doing too much at once.

"Take it easy." "Easy does it." "One day at a time." "Today is the first day of the rest of your life." "The journey of a thousand miles begins with one step." "Don't push the river." "Do unto others" ... I think you get the point.

There is a lot of good news here. It does not take the full "three miles in under an hour" to do the trick. If you are out of shape, or haven't exercised for some time, all you need to do is start. If you can only make it to the end of the block, then do that. Just start at a pace that seems brisk to you. Do not do so much that you get cramps and can't keep doing it regularly. Even if you can only walk one block when you start you will still get the beneficial effects. You will already be changing your metabolic rate. Your heart rate will increase and the process will already be starting to work.

As you get used to walking, add a little bit more to your time and distance. If you can only go a block the first time, next time try a to go that block plus maybe one or two more houses. After that work up to a block and a half, and so on. You don't have to do it all the first time out. Rome wasn't built in a day.

A general rule of thumb regarding exercise to stay safe and avoid injury is to aim toward increasing your exercise routine by 10% a week. You have the rest of your life in front of you. Start where you are, do what you can, and work up from there.

Probably the best news here is that taking a walk is actually quite pleasant, and it is a wonderful way to start or end the day.

Walking is a good time for thinking - or just the opposite - to take a break from thinking and the problems of the day. It's a perfect time for meditating. Also, contrary to some popular beliefs, exercise actually gives you energy rather than making you tired. You will be more energized and alert all day if you start with a walk.

Don't say to yourself, "I *have* to go exercise now." What fun is that? Instead, get excited. Say to yourself, "Hey, I get to go for a walk now! How nice! How pleasant! How lucky I am to get to go for a walk!"

Even if you are really dragging and the bed is cozy and it's drizzling outside and a million other reasons, it is only the first few steps that may be difficult. After that it really is quite pleasant to take a walk. Once you're out there it's easy.

I try to walk every day. And I tell myself that I am going to walk everyday. But I don't always make it. Instead, it turns out to be maybe five times per week. That is good enough as far as I am concerned. More would be better, but not that much better.

But walking doesn't have to be your thing. Any aerobic exercise will do: swimming, skiing, bicycling, dancing, skating, or using exercise equipment such as power-riders, treadmills, or rowing machines. And, of course, switching from one activity to another is fine. You just want to give your body the message that you intend to be an active person from now on.

You can even go ahead and join an aerobics class if you want! The idea is to just get started. Begin with a daily walk. After that, the sky is the limit. But do take it easy. Get medical clearance if you are uncertain about your capabilities. And have a nice walk.

But why don't I just skip eating a banana or two and not have to walk?

There used to be argument among researchers about the value of exercise in weight control. There were those who insisted it was a critical element to any program, and still others who claimed that if a person walked or ran a mile they would only be burning off about 100 calories exercise didn't play a major role in weight loss. You could just not eat a banana and reduce your calories by 100.

But the current research seems to show that aerobic exercise increases metabolism, both while you are doing the exercise and for an extended time after the exercise by "resetting" your overall metabolic rate.

EXERCISE REVIEW

Exercise is probably the number one determining factor in reaching and maintaining your weight goals. The DOWN-SIZER SYSTEM recommends that you do some aerobic exercise at least four times per week for a half an hour at a time. Remember, you do not have to join a gym to get results; moderate walking, swimming, or any activity that gets your heart rate up will increase your metabolism which is what burns - and thus reduces - fat.

A brisk walk is one of the best exercises available to us, and it is the kind of thing most of us can do our entire life, well into old age.

Also, keep in mind, it is easy and fun. The hardest part is the first step. After that it's easy!

DIET

Along with exercise, there are four basic principles in the DOWN-SIZER SYSTEM that are essential to weight control. They are eating a low-fat diet, paying attention to portion control, avoiding simple carbohydrates, and not skipping meals. Let's take these one at a time.

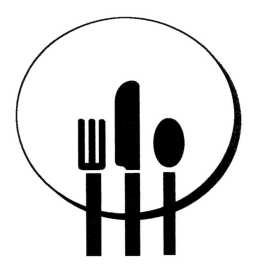

DOWN-SIZER
STEP #2

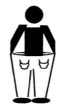

A LOW-FAT DIET

EAT UNDER 20 GRAMS OF FAT PER DAY

A low-fat diet is essential to losing and controlling your weight, as well as in promoting overall good health.

The average American diet contains approximately 75 - 80 grams of fat per day. The American Heart Association recommends eating under 30 grams of fat per day for optimum health. But in order to lose and control your weight, it is best to try to keep your fat grams to under 20 per day.

To do this, you will need to keep track of your daily intake of fat grams. Eating 20 grams of fat a day may be a drastic change for many of you. But it can be done, and it's not that hard to do. Once you start paying attention to the fat content in foods and learn which foods are high in fat and which are low in fat, it's not difficult to dramatically cut out a great deal of the fat you eat.

More and more low-fat and non-fat items are becoming available in the grocery stores all the time. Restaurants are also catching on to the demand and are beginning to offer menu items that are low in fat.

HOW DO YOU KNOW WHAT FOODS HAVE A LOT OF FAT IN THEM?

The best way to figure out the fat content of a food is to read the label. Most foods in the grocery stores have a nutrition labels which are easy to read. They list the fat content and other pertinent nutritional information of the food.

HOW TO READ A LABEL

Reading a nutrition label to determine the amount of fat per serving in a food is easy.

The first thing to do is look at the Total Fat content of the item. Total Fat content is listed about half way down on the left hand side of the label, followed by a number in grams (see illustration on next page).

Since you are trying to keep your fat intake to under 20 grams per day, it is not necessary to separate saturated fat from total fat.

The second thing you need to do is to determine the Serving Size. This important information is listed near the top of the label. The total fat content listed is in grams per serving. So, if the box (bottle, can, container, etc.) lists 5 servings per container, you will need to multiply the total fat grams by 5 to find out how much fat is in the whole package.

For example, if the Total Fat line reads 2 grams of fat, and the serving size reads 5 servings per container, the Total Fat in the entire package is 10 grams of fat (5 servings x 2 grams of fat per serving).

So, you can see it is essential that you read both the Total Fat content, as well as the number of servings per container. The Total Fat content is per serving, not per package.

Once you start reading labels and paying attention to the Fat Content in foods, you may be surprised at the amount of fat you will find in certain foods. Before I started paying attention to the Total Fat content in foods, I would grab a quick bite of cheese, or perhaps a spoonful of peanut butter if I was hungry, thinking it was healthy, full of good proteins, and generally harmless.

Little did I know that the cheese I was eating had about 8-10 grams of fat per ounce, and the peanut butter had about 8 grams per tablespoon!

What to look for when reading labels for __Total Fat Grams__ in foods.

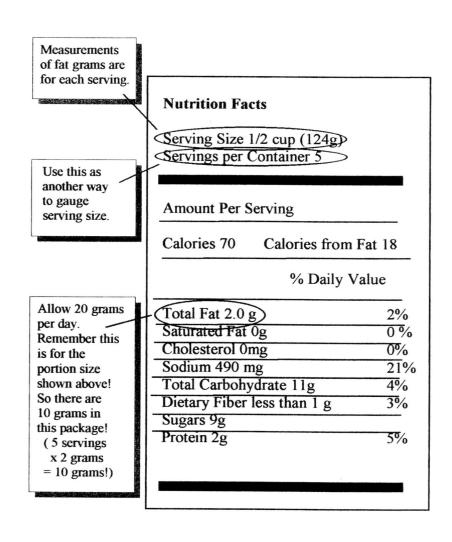

Measurements of fat grams are for each serving.

Use this as another way to gauge serving size.

Allow 20 grams per day. Remember this is for the portion size shown above! So there are 10 grams in this package!
(5 servings
 x 2 grams
 = 10 grams!)

Nutrition Facts

Serving Size 1/2 cup (124g)
Servings per Container 5

Amount Per Serving

Calories 70   Calories from Fat 18

% Daily Value

Total Fat 2.0 g	2%
Saturated Fat 0g	0 %
Cholesterol 0mg	0%
Sodium 490 mg	21%
Total Carbohydrate 11g	4%
Dietary Fiber less than 1 g	3%
Sugars 9g	
Protein 2g	5%

A couple bites of these foods has more fat than I should be eating all day. No wonder I was packing on the pounds. I was surprised to find out that there was a lot of fat in many cereals and snack crackers, and the seemingly innocuous blueberry muffin can have up to 30 grams of fat in one muffin! You'd be better off eating a fast food hamburger!

Some of the other foods I was surprised to find out about were sunflower seeds (14 grams per 1 oz.), mayonnaise (11-12 grams per tablespoon), salad dressings (8-10 grams per tablespoon), and guacamole (2 grams per tablespoon). If you have measured out anything to eat in terms of tablespoons, you will know that a tablespoon isn't very big. It is certainly easy to eat many tablespoons of guacamole at one sitting or to use many tablespoons of salad dressing on a salad.

You sit down with a nice garden salad and think you're doing something good for yourself and then drench it in salad dressing with more fat than you want to have all day.

The good news here is that again, the food manufacturers are catching on, and some very good non-fat salad dressings are now available. Just a short time ago the non-fat dressings all tasted terrible. But they have come a long way in a short time. If you have not tried any lately, give them another chance.

More good news is that most dairy products now have non-fat or low-fat alternatives. Many of the non-fat items are also actually quite good.

WHAT TO EAT AND NOT TO EAT, THAT IS THE QUESTION

You do not need to be a gourmet cook or spend hours in the kitchen everyday in order to start eating the right kinds of food. You can start with a few simple changes in your diet and add from there.

Most importantly, you need to find foods you like to eat, and you need to make preparing and eating new foods fun. If you make eating and cooking a chore, your new habits won't last any longer than an exercise routine you don't really like.

So what to do?

Of course, we all know fruits and vegetables are the best foods to eat for losing weight and gaining optimal health.

But that doesn't mean you have to go out today and become a vegetarian. Let's start simple and add from there.

Start by including more salads in your diet. Salads are easy to make, and you can easily vary them so you won't get too bored by eating the same thing over and over.

Start by adding salads to you meals. This will help fill you up, supply you with excellent foods, and increase your water intake as vegetables are generally high in water content. Plus, they will not add lots of fat into your diet.

In addition to adding salads to your diet, start using fruits as snacks. Have plenty around, cut them up, and make them easy to grab and snack on.

With a few exceptions, most fruits and vegetables are terrific. But stay away from avocados, they are full of fat. Whole grains and beans are also good foods. But avoid coconut, soybeans, peanuts and most other nuts. They are full of oil, i.e., fat.

Most meats are high in fat. However, a piece of steak about the size of your palm (around 4 oz.) with all the visible fat trimmed away will be in the neighborhood of about 8 grams of fat. It's possible to fit that into a low-fat diet.

Chicken is all right. Be sure to remove the skin before cooking since there is more fat in the skin than the rest of the chicken. A chicken breast contains about 4 grams of fat. The fat content in fish varies quite a bit, but in general you can eat a fair amount of fish in keeping with a low fat diet.

Hamburger is pretty much off the menu unless you get the 7% fat, or 5% fat. A little bit of meat can be worked into a low fat diet. Just read those labels.

Baked potatoes are good food. It is generally what gets put on them that causes the problem (butter, sour cream, bacon bits!). However, if you use non-fat butter substitutes and non-fat sour cream, you will be fine.

Throw away your frying pan. Get up. Go over to the kitchen right now. Throw it out! (Ok, so throwing it out might seem a little bit wasteful. Just put it away where you can not easily get to it.)

Don't use any kind of oil for cooking. Oil has approximately 14 grams of fat per tablespoon. Yikes! No frying allowed. Try instead to bake, grill, boil or broil.

Watch out for eggs. They have about 6 grams of fat per egg. The fat is all in the yoke. You can use egg substitutes (usually available in restaurants as well), which are often made up of just the whites of the eggs.

"Fast food" is generally "fat food." However, there are a few things on the menu at some of the fast food restaurants that could be worked in to a low-fat diet. Some of the grilled chicken sandwiches, for example, have in the neighborhood of 6 - 8 grams of fat. Order them without mayonnaise. And do not try to get away with eating fast food very often. It will quickly catch up with you. A large order of fries alone is around of 22 grams of fat. Ouch!

Regular potato chips are out. Ice cream, candy, and cookies are out. But, you know this already. (But can you cheat just a little? Yeah, sure, but just a little.)

Once you are aware of the fat content of certain foods it becomes difficult to enjoy them. You might ask yourself, "Is this donut really worth 20 grams of fat?" "Do I really need this bag of potato chips (10 grams/one ounce) or can I get by with some pretzels instead?" (Pretzels = no fat).

And how about dessert? Ice cream (10-25 grams of fat per scoop) vs. non-fat frozen yogurt (zero grams per scoop).

Many people actually prefer the taste of the lower fat content foods. After eating a lower fat diet for awhile, I find that if I drink a glass of whole milk now, I practically gag. Fried foods make my stomach hurt. And rich cream and oil sauces are simply too rich for me to eat. They don't even taste good anymore.

WHAT ABOUT UNLABELED FOODS?

Fortunately most vegetables and fruits have very little fat in them so you do not have to worry. You can eat pretty much as many of these things as you'd like.

You might want to get one of the small "fat counter" books on the market. These books are available in many bookstores and grocerystores. (There is also a fat and calorie list at the end of this book.) These books and lists will let you know the fat content of unlabeled foods.

CONCLUSION

There are many fine foods to eat. You do not have to be a vegetarian or eat a macrobiotic diet or stick to a certain diet book's regime or buy special foods.

It is important to understand the concept of eating low-fat, and then the job (and the fun) is finding foods you like to eat. If you are just following a set of rules, it is difficult to stick with making changes in your diet and lifestyle. Once your inspiration is gone, usually the diet goes, too.

Instead of mapping out a diet for you, it is important that you find things you like to eat and want to eat, so you can begin to eat them for the rest of your life.

You are starting a new way of living, not just another diet. You are learning new ways to eat. You are finding new foods you like and are getting rid of some foods you don't want in your diet anymore.

It can be exciting to find new foods and new ways of preparing them. This is the beginning of something fresh. Something long lasting, and a new direction. Get excited. This can be fun.

Pay attention to what you are eating.

If you are like many of us, we sit down to eat and begin reading the paper or talking or watching TV or doing some other distracting activity. We often eat without really paying attention to what we are doing. We might be half way through our meal before we even notice it or really taste it. It's no wonder so many of us tend to overeat. One way to avoid this is to pay attention to what you are eating right from the beginning of a meal. Pay attention to how good something tastes or how satisfying it is. Do this in the beginning of the meal instead of waiting until you're almost finished with it. You can eat a lot less this way, and you will enjoy your meals more as well.

LOW-FAT REVIEW

Read those labels and keep the fat grams to under 20 per grams per day. Remember, the amount of fat listed on the label is per serving. Always check to see what constitutes a "serving size."

DOWN-SIZER STEP #3
PORTION CONTROL

How much we eat really does make a difference in terms of losing or gaining weight. This seems simple enough. But it is sometimes hard to know just how much to eat.

In the real world it is difficult to count calories or weigh your food or do some of the other "tricks" you may have learned or heard about for keeping portion size within reasonable limits.

It is possible to do some of these things for a while, especially when you first start and are motivated and excited. But it is almost impossible to maintain weighing and counting and calculating your food intake. It just doesn't work that well over the long term.

Instead, try the "handful" method. The "handful" measure is a convenient way to estimate how much to eat. It is a method you can actually use without too much trouble.

The way you apply the handful idea is this: Imagine if you can, fitting the food that is on your plate in one hand. If your meal could fit on one hand you are in good shape.

For most people roughly 4 handfuls of food per day is about right. This will vary, of course, depending on the size of your hand. (If you have small hands, you can handle a little more, maybe 5 or 6 handfuls per day.)

Some good news here is this rule does not apply to green vegetables or fruits. You can have all of those you want.

Using this method should result in your eating about 1100 to 1200 calories a day. This is not a starvation diet by far, but one in which you will lose weight at a reasonable pace.

A "handful" of food is a meal. The measurements will not be exact, but weighing and counting are not exact measures either.

And, besides, it is not really necessary to be exact anyway. We are not able to measure exercise, temperature, and other factors exactly either. Instead, we just need a rule, or a tool, that will keep us more or less on track.

The handful method is inexact, but it is a useful tool for guessing at appropriate portions. Once you reach your goal weight you may be able to eat more food or larger portions.

PORTION CONTROL REVIEW

Use portion control. Don't try to weigh your food or count your calories, remember the handful idea. For people with relatively normal size hands eat up to four handfuls of food per day.

A handful is about as much food as you could actually place on your open hand.

TAKE AIM!

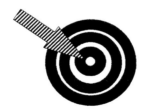

Have a goal weight. It is easier to hit a target if you know what it is you are aiming at.

Variations in your weight.

It is sometimes surprising - but true - that one's weight can vary as much as four or five pounds over the course of a day or a month. Weight can be effected by menstrual cycles, sodium in your diet, and other factors. Your weight in the morning will be different than your weight just after you eat lunch. It is important not to get too hung up on these variations.

If after reaching your goal you begin to see a trend toward putting weight back on, you are probably eating too much. If you hop on the scale and see it start to move up you may want to pay more attention to portion size that day. If you are at, or under, your goal weight you can relax a bit more about it.

However, try not to let your weight sneak up beyond five pounds over your goal or target weight. If it does, it is probably time too get serious again about portion control.

Many people simply have to pay close attention to their portion size on an ongoing basis. But again, it's easier than you might think.

A Quick Five Pounds

Salt in a person's diet tends to make them bloat, retain water, and generally be heavier. If you want to drop a quick five pounds the easiest way to do it is to watch how much salt (sodium) you take in. It won't have much effect on your overall weight loss, and will have little effect in the long run, but it shouldn't cause any problems, and there may well be other health reasons to limit your salt intake as well.

Nobody's Friend...the Wight Scale!

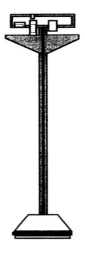

All scales are going to read a little bit different. Even the high-tech scales used in doctors offices all read a little bit different. If you go to three different doctors this week, chances are you will have three different weights. And your bathroom scale may read several pounds different from your doctor's. In order to avoid confusion and disappointment, it might be useful just to find a scale you are comfortable using and to weigh yourself consistently at the same time of day.

Don't get too caught up in the numbers. Just get a base reading and try to get the readings to move in the right directions. That is, you want the numbers to start moving down the scale from where you started.

DOWN-SIZER STEP #4
Do Not Skip Meals

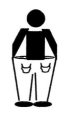

It may seem odd that a book on becoming a DOWN-SIZER would suggest not skipping meals. It would stand to reason that eating less often would be a good idea. Wouldn't you be just that much better off if you could skip a meal now and then? While this sounds logical, it turns out that it's not quite that simple.

When we skip meals, our bodies start to think, "Oh-oh, there must not be any food around. I better slow down my metabolism and squirrel away whatever food I do get for a rainy day."

Your body then lowers your metabolism, doing the opposite of what it does when you exercise. So, the food you eat later in the day, instead of being used for energy, will tend to be stored away as fat.

So, it is important to eat at least three meals a day. Eating four times a day is also fine. And if you still watch total portions, even more frequent meals are OK.

Since we do not want our bodies to go think we are starving and therefore slow down our metabolism, it is important that we eat breakfast. For some people this is especially difficult. Some people have an aversion to eating first thing in the morning. It also seems to be the easiest meal for most people to skip.

But try to eat at least a little something for breakfast. This will inform your body that you are not indeed starving today, and it can feel free to burn up your fat for energy today.

It is good to eat some protein (cottage cheese, non-fat milk, egg substitutes, yogurt, most instant breakfast drinks) in the morning. This gets your metabolism back on track after fasting overnight.

For those of you who can't stand the thought of eating in the morning or if you're just in a hurry, one solution is to use the drinkable form of Knox Gelatin. Knox Gelatin is almost a pure protein powder and it is available in the Jello (etc.) aisle at the grocery store. It is generally orange flavored. There is also an unflavored version, which can be mixed with water, low-fat milk, or some other liquid. Or you might want to try some protein powders from your local health food store. It is easy to drink, and has what your body needs to kick start your metabolism for the day.

And, as mentioned above, many of the instant breakfast drinks are also excellent ways to start the day.

In short, regular meals with reasonable eating habits are the best and easiest route to weight control.

DO NOT SKIP MEALS REVIEW

When we skip meals our bodies tend to slow down and conserve energy. It does so by holding on to fat. Skipping meals will ultimately lower our metabolism, doing the opposite of what happens when we exercise. What that means is that the food you eat later in the same day, instead of being used for energy, will tend to be squirreled away into fat. So it's important to eat at least three meals a day. Four is also fine. And if you still watch total portions, even more frequent meals are fine.

Eating regular meals with reasonable eating habits is the best and easiest route to weight control.

DOWN-SIZER STEP #5

Avoid Simple Carbohydrates, Refined Sugars, and Over Processed Foods.

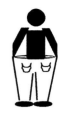

There are three kinds - or categories - of foods. All foods are either proteins, carbohydrates, or fats. Carbohydrates are basically the sugars and starches.

The simple carbohydrates, refined sugars, and over processed foods include sugar you might find in a number of places (cakes, cookies, ice cream, candy, grapes, raisins, alcohol, etc.), white breads (including French bread and sourdough), and white rice.

The major problem with these foods is that they actually make you feel hungry. That's right. Eating the simple carbohydrates and refined sugars will actually make you more hungry than if you ate nothing at all.

How does this happen?

Basically, simple carbohydrates, the refined sugars, and over processed foods, cause problems because they mess with the insulin in your system, as well as raising and lowering your blood sugar.

Insulin is a hormone secreted by the pancreas in response to ingesting (eating) any food. It speeds up and assists your metabolism in digesting your food. However, the simple carbohydrates and over processed sugars are so refined that they do not need to use the insulin that has been produced. So the insulin runs around wondering what to do with itself. It has been stimulated so you must have eaten something. If not, get something down here so we have something to do. Ahh, a feeling of hunger!

Also, these foods end up leaving you with low blood sugar. This happens about a half an hour or so after you eat these foods. People with low blood sugar also tend to have a feeling of hunger.

So, if you eat these foods, you will actually stimulate your hunger. Eating these things will make you feel hungrier than if you hadn't eaten anything at all. Odd, isn't it?

You can see this principle in action fairly easily. For example, you may be familiar with the notion that people are often hungry again an hour after eating in a Chinese restaurant, and you might wonder why. A lot of the classic Chinese foods you will find in most Chinese restaurants are actually very healthy and filling. The chicken, vegetables and other foods commonly found in Chinese dishes are quite nourishing. It is the white rice is running through your system so quickly - bypassing the insulin - that stimulates your hunger. When you eat rice, use brown rice. It will not have the same effect as white rice.

Another example of this process can be found in the the custom of many restaurants that serve a basket full of white bread or bread sticks before the main meal. Have you ever noticed you can eat a lot of bread before your meal arrives and still have room for the main course? If the bread actually filled you up, this tradition of serving bread before meals wouldn't survive. It would put restaurants out of business.

This is a strange concept, I know. And it surprises a lot of people, but I invite you to try it out yourself. Have a little ice cream and watch. If you are like most people you will notice that in about a half an hour or so you will start to feel a little hungry again.

If you go back for just a little more ice cream to satisfy your hunger you will find yourself getting hungry again shortly after that. If this keeps up you might find yourself going round and round with the ice cream carton all night.

Sometimes eating something sour will take away the craving for sweets. Next time you're craving a sweet, try a bit of something sour and see if it doesn't change your direction. It might just make the difference.

An all too familiar - and counter productive - pattern.

All too often skipping meals and eating the simple carbohydrates and refined sugars go together.

Many people skip breakfast. After all, aren't we trying to eat less and lose weight? It's fairly easy for many people to avoid eating breakfast, and they are under the mistaken assumption that skipping a meal will be good for losing weight.

Sometimes, people are truly inspired and still ambitious at lunch time, so they are able to eat a small lunch or skip it altogether.

But as the day, and our ambition, start to wane, it is now dinner time. If we should happen to overeat a little bit, which is easy to do by this point, we may feel uncomfortably full after dinner. Sometimes a dessert will take away that stuffed feeling. So we have a little something sweet. We may then feel a little better, but low and behold about twenty minutes later we're hungry again.

This is when the binge eating starts. We decide to have a little snack. All too often the snack includes a simple carbohydrate and/or refined sugar product. All too often the snack is just not all that healthy and is full of sugar. We eat it, and end up making ourselves hungry again. So we eat a little something else. It's easy to keep this up all evening.

Maybe we convince ourselves that we'll make up for it tomorrow. In fact, we'll start by not eating breakfast!

We end up eating more throughout the evening than we would have if we'd eaten reasonably throughout the day. In addition, since we skipped meals, we convinced our body that we should slow down our metabolism and store our fat for a rainy day instead of burning it for energy today.

The Solution

The solution to this problem is simple. Here's what to do:

1) Eat normally at breakfast and lunch so you are not unusually hungry at dinner time.

2) Pay attention and don't over eat in the evening.

3) If you do feel full, just go ahead and feel full for awhile. Resist the temptation to eat the dessert. Wait for a length of time before eating anything else.

4) If you still feel a need for a snack later in the evening, have something with some protein in it. This will make you feel satiated so you can stop as opposed to eating the simple carbohydrates which will send you round and round the cycle discussed above.

It is important to control the evening binges if you are going to control your weight. If the above evening scenario does apply to you, see if you can find a way to interrupt it.

Remember, try to avoid skipping meals and avoid the simple carbohydrates.

Avoid Simple Carbohydrates, Refined Sugars, and Over Processed Foods Review

Starches, sugars, cakes, white bread, white rice, grapes, alcohol, etc., all effect your insulin level and blood sugar and end up stimulating your hunger. They actually make you more hungry than if you'd eaten nothing at all.

How Much Weight Can I Lose and How Fast?

People frequently want to know how much and how fast they can expect to lose weight. This is a reasonable question, and, of course, the answer depends on how diligently one works at it.

A reasonable amount to expect might be 2 pounds per week, or maybe 10 pounds per month. Losing weight at this rate will give you time to implement your new lifestyle and eating habits and will help you keep from putting the weight right back on once you've lost it.

Sometimes the more weight you have to lose, the faster it will come off. If you have just a few pounds to lose, it may happen at a slower rate.

But how much and how fast might be the wrong questions to ask. Don't think of this as a diet or a short term quick fix. This book and the principles within are about a way to live. A lifestyle. This lifestyle is not something you will do for a little while until you reach your weight goals. Instead it is a way to live, to eat, and to exercise for the rest of your life.

But also, don't think of this "lifestyle change" as some large and looming task. If you start thinking about changing forever, it can look like a daunting task. Think of it this way. You're not going on a diet; you are simply giving up certain foods and habits and are replacing them with others.

Also, take it day by day. One day at a time. Easy does it, and all the rest. If you say to yourself, "I can never eat a donut or piece of chocolate again for the rest of my life," you may well be tempted too put several pieces in your mouth immediately. And who could blame you?

Break this process down into steps you can actually achieve. Make it easy for yourself to succeed. Don't think too far in the future. Just take it day by day - meal by meal - or hour by hour. Soon it will be easy.

You are developing a change in you habits and are creating a new direction for your life.

Instead of asking how fast and how much, better questions might include; How to get started? What are some good books to read? What else can I add to these ideas? Why have I put this off so long? And when should I start?

The answer to the latter, of course, is right now.

This is your body we're talking about. Your habits. Your lifestyle. This is your life. The best question of all may be "What are you going to do with it?"

The principles in this book really work. You can always learn more information, do more exercise, and gain more knowledge than we have discussed; but if you apply what we have discussed and if you put the principles in to action, you can - and will - begin to lose and control your weight.

The ultimate answer is yes. *Yes, you can!*

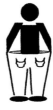

Congratulations!

You're on your way.

2

REVIEW

How to become a Down-Sizer!

The Essentials of the 5 Point Plan for Weight Control

1. Eat a low-fat diet. Read the labels on your food, and keep the fat grams you eat to under 20 per day.

2. Exercise. Aim for walking three miles in under an hour, four times per week. But start with going for a walk. Remember, you don't have to join a gym to get results. Any activity that gets your heart rate up (walking, bicycling, power riders, swimming, dancing, etc.) will increase your metabolism, which, in turn, will burn fat.

3. Use portion control. Use the handful idea. A handful is about as much food as you could actually place on your open hand.

4. Don't skip meals. Skipping meals sends your
body into a starvation/conservation mode.
This lowers metabolism and makes your
body hold onto fat instead of using it
for energy. Regular meals with reasonable
eating habits is the best and easiest route
to weight control.

5. Avoid simple carbohydrates and refined sugars.

They stimulate your hunger and actually make
you more hungry than if you had eaten nothing
at all.

3

101 *Ideas*

on the Subject

1. Remind yourself that yes, you can do this!
2. Fast foods = fat foods.
3. What happened before - in the past - does not mean that is the way it will be today or tomorrow.
4. Do not use oil of any kind.
5. Be a dreamer.
6. Limit your fat intake to 20 grams or less per day.
7. Yes is the answer!
8. Eat a lot of salads and check out the stores for non-fat salad dressings. There are some pretty good ones out there.
9. If at first you don't succeed...

> Remind yourself that you are
> not on a diet.
> You are developing a new lifestyle.

10. Don't give up on yourself; believe in yourself. Say out loud "Yes I can!" Mean it! Believe it!

11. The journey of a thousand miles begins with one step.
12. When you can, use the stairs instead of the escalator. Walk when you can instead of riding. Be an active person. Think like an active person.
13. Find a walking buddy or a friend to exercise with.
14. Go to the window, and yell, "I'm mad as hell and I'm not going to take it anymore!"
15. Control how much alcohol you drink. It will stimulate hunger and lower your ability to control your inhibitions, including control over your eating habits.

> Reward yourself with something other than food.
> Buy yourself a magazine, new clothes, music
> or flowers. Take a walk in the park.
> Give yourself a pat on the back.
> What else can you think of? Be creative!

16. Make interesting foods and snacks.
17. Remember the handful method and the idea of portion control. About a Handful of food is a meal for most people. Eat up to four handfuls of food per day.
18. Learn one new recipe per week. Soon you'll have many to choose from.
19. Don't shop when you are hungry. If you've ever done this, you know that suddenly everything looks good. Take the time to buy the right foods.
20. Drink some water before meals. This helps you feel fuller faster.
21. Drink 6-8 glasses of water a day. This will help flush your system.
22. Chew slowly, pay attention to what you are eating, and don't just eat on automatic pilot.
23. Eat - or drink - some protein for breakfast.

24. Avoid fried foods.

25. Even though there are people starving in some places in the world, it is still not necessary to clean your plate. Feel free to contribute in other ways.

> ## Cravings Pass.
> ## Give yourself a few minutes
> ## before giving in.

26. Eat to live; do not live to eat.

27. You don't have to keep eating just because it tastes good.

28. Donate your frying pan to someone skinny.

29. If you are used to snacking while you watch TV, try to break the habit. Just say no! Be here now! Or find some other catch phrase to help you remember that you are starting fresh and are heading toward a new life released from the bounds of compulsive behavior. Start from here and move forward. Find new habits.

30. Why do you think they call it junk food?

31. Pickles will help take away a "sweet tooth."

> ## Eat when you are hungry.
> ## Don't eat because you are bored or
> ## depressed or lonely. Accept and
> ## deal with your feelings.

32. Avoid grapes and raisins. They are like little packets of sugar and will end up making you feel hungry.

33. When you do snack, eat low calorie foods and fruits without a lot of sugar or fat.

34. Eat fruits: apples, bananas, blackberries, cantaloupe and all of the melons, grapefruit, lemons, oranges, peaches, pears, fresh and unsweetened canned pineapple, raspberries, strawberries and tomatoes.

> Persistence is the key ingredient
> that separates those who succeed from those
> who fail. Don't give up on yourself.
> Say out loud, "Yes, I can!" Mean it. Believe it.
> Get excited...you're on your way!

35. Save the money you would have spent on buying candy or donuts for a week and buy yourself a present instead.
36. Avoid peanuts and other nuts. They are full of fat.
37. Spices are generally OK, but do not use butter. There are some good butter substitutes out there. Try them out.
38. Keep apple slices, chopped carrots, and other snack foods ready and at hand so you can grab them instead of reaching for the bag of chips or the cookie jar. (What are you doing with a cookie jar anyway?!)
39. Eat vegetables. Artichokes, asparagus, beans, beets, broccoli, Brussels sprouts, cabbage, carrots, cauliflower, celery, cucumbers, eggplant, endive, green peas, lettuce, mushrooms, onions, parsnips, potatoes, radishes, spinach, squash, string beans, Swiss chard, turnips...just to name a few.
40. Don't skip meals, especially breakfast. Eating regular meals at regular times is essential to controlling your weight.
41. If you crave something sweet, try something sour or spicy instead. Strong flavors will often get rid of the craving for something sweet.

42. Eat protein: Lean portions of beef, lamb and calves' liver, Egg Beaters, poultry (with skin removed before cooking), fish, seafood, non-fat milk, non-fat cheeses, non-fat yogurt and non-fat cottage cheese, lentils and beans (but not soy beans).

43. Remember, cravings pass in a few minutes.

44. A clear soup is a good soup. Avoid creamed, canned and restaurant soups. They are generally high in fat. Buy fat-free soups.

45. Read the labels. Read the labels. Read the labels.

46. Use brown rice instead of white rice.

47. Pasta is OK. Just watch out for the sauces. Read the label. Don't add a lot of fat to homemade sauces.

48. Picture yourself at your ideal weight. Keep the image in mind and begin to act, move, and feel like you will feel when you reach your goal.

49. Don't make excuses for overeating. If you are bored or depressed or whatever, you don't have to reach for food. Take a walk. Plan a fun night out. Start a support group with friends. Join Overeaters Anonymous. There are many things you can do that do not include eating. What are some others?

Do what is necessary today. Tomorrow will take care of itself.

---

50. A rhyme for good eating: Don't fry
instead broil
grill, bake
or boil.

51. Use smaller plates. This will help you eat smaller portions.
52. An apple a day keeps some fat grams away.
53. Do not think of your new eating habits as a "diet." Instead, think of it as a new lifelong, good health program. This is not a temporary diet. This is the beginning of your new life!
54. Exercise. Find something you like to do. Exercise will actually give you more energy, and it feels great to start getting in shape. Don't overdo it. Just start.
55. If you crave a particular food over and over, it is possible that you have developed an addiction to that food. Try to eat this food only once every few days. You may be able to break the habit.
56. Don't let other people's opinions, ideas, criticisms or disapproval manipulate you. You do not need to justify your behavior or explain reasons for your diet or your desire to control your weight. People often oppose change in themselves and in those around them. Of course, it is worthwhile to listen to - and seriously consider - genuine concerns from those around you, but it is your life...listen to your heart and inner wisdom.

> **Set a clear goal weight that you would like to reach. It is much easier to hit a target if you know what you are aiming at.**

57. Give yourself a break. Don't be too hard on yourself. Don't beat yourself up if you cheat now and then. Don't feel guilty and use that as an excuse to binge. Instead, give yourself credit for all you have done right.

58. Keep a positive attitude. A slip doesn't have to be a fall. And a fall doesn't have to keep you down. Get up, shake off, and move forward. Remember falling off your bicycle when you were learning? Just get up and try it again.

59. Air popped popcorn is ok! Just forget the salt and butter.

> Maintain a positive attitude.
> A slip doesn't have to be a fall.
> And a fall doesn't have to keep you down.

60. If you drink milk, work your way step by step from whole milk to non-fat. At first you might notice the difference from whole to 2% to 1% etc., but pretty soon non-fat milk will taste like just the real thing.

61. Salty foods make you retain water.

62. Post your ideal weight in an obvious place.

63. Don't become obsessed with your weight and the reading on the scale. Just get a base reading and then get the numbers to start going down from there. Every scale measures a little differently and people's weight can fluctuate through the day, week, and month.

64. Remember these five things: exercise, eat under 20 grams of fat per day, use portion control (the handful method), avoid simple carbohydrates, and don't skip meals. This is just about all you need to know!

> Take a Walk...It's Fun! Don't say to yourself
> "I have to exercise now." What fun is that?
> Instead, get excited. Say to yourself, "Hey!
> I get to go for a walk now! How nice.
> How pleasant. How lucky I am!"

65. If you are overweight, you probably have a genetic predisposition to being so.
66. Developing a new lifestyle is easier than you may think.
67. Exercise is fun.
68. Find some good books to hang out with.
69. Find someone who lost weight and kept it off; do what they did.
70. But, remember to be yourself. Find your own path. Do what makes sense for you.
71. Fat contains about twice as many calories as carbohydrates and proteins.
72. Rome wasn't built in a day. Results take time. But make steady progress in the right direction.
73. Don't be afraid to ask for help.
74. Talk it over with your family doctor.
75. Talk if over with a psychotherapist.
76. Keep your goals in mind and take daily action - even if only very small steps - toward those goals.
77. Every time you step on a scale and it hasn't gone up, you are doing well.
78. If you step on a scale and the numbers have gone up, don't give up, just get back to basics.
79. Don't worry. Be happy. You don't have to look like a Barbie doll to be happy.

Decide. Decide that you want to live a new life and make the commitment to that new life a reality. Today, make it your intention, your stated goal, that from this moment forth, you intend to have the life you want to have.

80. You don't have to lose weight if you don't want to.

81. Health risks of being overweight include being a major contributing factors in premature heart disease, arthritis, depression, breast cancer, prostrate cancer, hypertension, diabetes, and a variety of other ailments and diseases.

82. If not now, when?

Yes is the answer!

83. Sometimes, as you begin to exercise, you may lose fat but gain muscle. Don't get too hung up on the numbers on the scale. Pay more attention to how you feel and how your clothes fit.

84. Imagine!

85. Aim toward increasing your exercise routine by 10% per week until you get to your goal program.

86. As you begin changing your life, there may be hurdles, slips, and falls along the way. But keep going. Perseverance will get the job done. Don't let anything stop you or hinder your resolve.

87. If you are overweight, it does not mean that you have a psychological problem.

88. Begin implementing your new healthy lifestyle today.

89. Every day in every way, I'm getting better and better.

90. I think I can. I think I can.

91. Aerobic means air, or more specifically oxygen in the air. Exercise "with air."

92. Try cross country skiing, downhill skiing, jumping rope, dancing, swimming, jumping on mini trampolines, walking, hiking, taking a row boat ride, using a stationary bicycle, taking a bike ride, roller skating, ice skating.

93. Believe in yourself.
94. Whether you think you can or whether you think you can't, you are probably right.
95. It's your life. Take control of it.
96. Just because you are craving something doesn't mean you have to eat it.
97. As you lose weight, you will gain energy.
98. Losing weight is good for your blood pressure.
99. There must be about a million good recipe books out there.
100. Don't be afraid to ask your doctor questions. Also, don't be afraid to question your doctor's answers.

101. *Today* *is the first day of the rest of your life!*

4

1200 Cal Day

20 gram Fat per Day

No papes

DOWN-SIZER

Calorie and
Fat Gram Chart
of 1000 Foods

Raw data provided by the
U.S. department of Agriculture

No mayo

Organized by and available online at
http://www.caloriecountercharts.com

3½ meat - 8½ gr

No avacado - 30 gr Fat

Low Dressing

No Butter

Low Fat Cheese

Pasta - Moderation

Alphabetical Listing of Foods

Description of food		Fat (grams)	Food Energy (calories)
1000 ISLAND, SALAD DRSNG, LOCAL	1 TBSP	2	25
1000 ISLAND, SALAD DRSNG, REGLR	1 TBSP	6	60
100% NATURAL CEREAL	1 OZ	6	135
40% BRAN FLAKES, KELLOGG'S	1 OZ	1	90
40% BRAN FLAKES, POST	1 OZ	0	90
ALFALFA SEEDS, SPROUTED, RAW	1 CUP	0	10
ALL-BRAN CEREAL	1 OZ	1	70
ALMONDS, SLIVERED	1 CUP	70	795
ALMONDS, WHOLE	1 OZ	15	165
ANGELFOOD CAKE, FROM MIX	1 CAKE	2	1510
ANGELFOOD CAKE, FROM MIX	1 PIECE	0	125
APPLE JUICE, CANNED	1 CUP	0	115
APPLE PIE	1 PIE	105	2420
APPLE PIE	1 PIECE	18	405
APPLESAUCE, CANNED, SWEETENED	1 CUP	0	195
APPLESAUCE, CANNED, UNSWEETENED	1 CUP	0	105
APPLES, DRIED, SULFURED	10 RINGS	0	155
APPLES, RAW, PEELED, SLICED	1 CUP	0	65
APPLES, RAW, UNPEELED, 2 PER LB	1 APPLE	1	125
APPLES, RAW, UNPEELED, 3 PER LB	1 APPLE	0	80
APRICOT NECTAR, NO ADDED VIT C	1 CUP	0	140
APRICOTS, CANNED, JUICE PACK	1 CUP	0	120
APRICOTS, CANNED, JUICE PACK	3 HALVES	0	40
APRICOTS, DRIED, COOKED, UNSWTN	1 CUP	0	210
APRICOTS, DRIED, UNCOOKED	1 CUP	1	310
APRICOTS, RAW	3 APRCOT	0	50
APRICOT, CANNED, HEAVY SYRUP	1 CUP	0	215
APRICOT, CANNED, HEAVY SYRUP	3 HALVES	0	70
ARTICHOKES, GLOBE, COOKED, DRN	1 ARTCHK	0	55
ASPARAGUS, CKD FRM FRZ, DRN, CUT	1 CUP	1	50
ASPARAGUS, CKD FRM FRZ, DR, SPER	4 SPEARS	0	15
ASPARAGUS, CKD FRM RAW, DR, CUT	1 CUP	1	45
ASPARAGUS, CKD FRM RAW, DR, SPER	4 SPEARS	0	15
ASPARAGUS, CANNED, SPEARS, NOSALT	4 SPEARS	0	10

Description of food		Fat (grams)	Food Energy (calories)
ASPARAGUS,CANNED,SPEARS,W/SALT	4 SPEARS	0	10
AVOCADOS, CALIFORNIA	1 AVOCDO	30	305
AVOCADOS, FLORIDA	1 AVOCDO	27	340
BAGELS, EGG	1 BAGEL	2	200
BAGELS, PLAIN	1 BAGEL	2	200
BAKING POWDER, LOW SODIUM	1 TSP	0	5
BAKING POWDER, STRGHT PHOSPHAT	1 TSP	0	5
BAKING POWDER,SAS, CA PO4	1 TSP	0	5
BAKING POWDER,SAS,CAPO4+CASO4	1 TSP	0	5
BAKING PWDR BISCUITS,FROM MIX	1 BISCUT	3	95
BAKING PWDR BISCUITS,HOMERECPE	1 BISCUT	5	100
BAKING PWDR BISCUITS,REFRGDOGH	1 BISCUT	2	65
BAMBOO SHOOTS, CANNED, DRAINED	1 CUP	1	25
BANANAS	1 BANANA	1	105
BANANAS, SLICED	1 CUP	1	140
BARBECUE SAUCE	1 TBSP	0	10
BARLEY, PEARLED,LIGHT, UNCOOKD	1 CUP	2	700
BEAN SPROUTS, MUNG, COOKD,DRAN	1 CUP	0	25
BEAN SPROUTS, MUNG, RAW	1 CUP	0	30
BEAN WITH BACON SOUP, CANNED	1 CUP	6	170
BEANS,DRY,CANNED,W/FRANKFURTER	1 CUP	18	365
BEANS,DRY,CANNED,W/PORK+SWTSCE	1 CUP	12	385
BEANS,DRY,CANNED,W/PORK+TOMSCE	1 CUP	7	310
BEEF AND VEGETABLE STEW,HM RCP	1 CUP	11	220
BEEF BROTH, BOULLN, CONSM,CNND	1 CUP	1	15
BEEF GRAVY, CANNED	1 CUP	5	125
BEEF HEART, BRAISED	3 OZ	5	150
BEEF LIVER, FRIED	3 OZ	7	185
BEEF NOODLE SOUP, CANNED	1 CUP	3	85
BEEF POTPIE, HOME RECIPE	1 PIECE	30	515
BEEF ROAST, EYE O RND, LEAN	2.6 OZ	5	135
BEEF ROAST, EYE O RND,LEAN+FAT	3 OZ	12	205
BEEF ROAST, RIB, LEAN ONLY	2.2 OZ	9	150
BEEF ROAST, RIB, LEAN + FAT	3 OZ	26	315
BEEF STEAK,SIRLOIN,BROIL,LEAN	2.5 OZ	6	150
BEEF STEAK,SIRLOIN,BROIL,LN+FT	3 OZ	15	240
BEEF, CANNED, CORNED	3 OZ	10	185

Description of food		Fat (grams)	Food Energy (calories)
BEEF, CKD,BTTM ROUND,LEAN ONLY	2.8 OZ	8	175
BEEF, CKD,BTTM ROUND,LEAN+ FAT	3 OZ	13	220
BEEF, CKD,CHUCK BLADE,LEANONLY	2.2 OZ	9	170
BEEF, CKD,CHUCK BLADE,LEAN+FAT	3 OZ	26	325
BEEF, DRIED, CHIPPED	2.5 OZ	4	145
BEER, LIGHT	12 FL OZ	0	95
BEER, REGULAR	12 FL OZ	0	150
BEET GREENS, COOKED, DRAINED	1 CUP	0	40
BEETS, CANNED, DRAINED,NO SALT	1 CUP	0	55
BEETS, CANNED, DRAINED,W/ SALT	1 CUP	0	55
BEETS, COOKED, DRAINED, DICED	1 CUP	0	55
BEETS, COOKED, DRAINED, WHOLE	2 BEETS	0	30
BLACK-EYED PEAS, DRY, COOKED	1 CUP	1	190
BLACK BEANS, DRY, COOKED,DRAN	1 CUP	1	225
BLACKBERRIES, RAW	1 CUP	1	75
BLACKEYE PEAS, IMMATR,RAW,CKED	1 CUP	1	180
BLACKEYE PEAS,IMMTR,FRZN,CKED	1 CUP	1	225
BLUE CHEESE	1 OZ	8	100
BLUE CHEESE SALAD DRESSING	1 TBSP	8	75
BLUEBERRIES, FROZEN, SWEETENED	1 CUP	0	185
BLUEBERRIES, FROZEN, SWEETENED	10 OZ	0	230
BLUEBERRIES, RAW	1 CUP	1	80
BLUEBERRY MUFFINS, HOME RECIPE	1 MUFFIN	5	135
BLUEBERRY MUFFINS,FROM COM MIX	1 MUFFIN	5	140
BLUEBERRY PIE	1 PIE	102	2285
BLUEBERRY PIE	1 PIECE	17	380
BOLOGNA	2 SLICES	16	180
BOSTON BROWN BREAD,W/WHTECRNM	1 SLICE	1	95
BOSTON BROWN BREAD,W/YLLWCRNML	1 SLICE	1	95
BOUILLON, DEHYDRTD, UNPREPARED	1 PKT	1	15
BRAN MUFFINS, FROM COMMERL MIX	1 MUFFIN	4	140
BRAN MUFFINS, HOME RECIPE	1 MUFFIN	6	125
BRAUNSCHWEIGER	2 SLICES	18	205
BRAZIL NUTS	1 OZ	19	185
BREAD STUFFING,FROM MX,DRYTYPE	1 CUP	31	500
BREAD STUFFING,FROM MX,MOIST	1 CUP	26	420
BREADCRUMBS, DRY, GRATED	1 CUP	5	390

Description of food		Fat (grams)	Food Energy (calories)
BROCCOLI, FRZN, COOKED, DRANED	1 CUP	0	50
BROCCOLI, FRZN, COOKED, DRANED	1 PIECE	0	10
BROCCOLI, RAW	1 SPEAR	1	40
BROCCOLI, RAW, COOKED, DRAINED	1 CUP	0	45
BROCCOLI, RAW, COOKED, DRAINED	1 SPEAR	1	50
BROWN AND SERVE SAUSAGE, BRWND	1 LINK	5	50
BROWN GRAVY FROM DRY MIX	1 CUP	2	80
BROWNIES W/ NUTS, FRM HOME RECP	1 BROWNE	6	95
BROWNIES W/ NUTS, FRSTNG, CMMRCL	1 BROWNE	4	100
BRUSSELS SPROUTS, FRZN, COOKED	1 CUP	1	65
BRUSSELS SPROUTS, RAW, COOKED	1 CUP	1	60
BUCKWHEAT FLOUR, LIGHT, SIFTED	1 CUP	1	340
BULGUR, UNCOOKED	1 CUP	3	600
BUTTERMILK, DRIED	1 CUP	7	465
BUTTERMILK, FLUID	1 CUP	2	100
BUTTER, SALTED	1 PAT	4	35
BUTTER, SALTED	1 TBSP	11	100
BUTTER, SALTED	1/2 CUP	92	810
BUTTER, UNSALTED	1 PAT	4	35
BUTTER, UNSALTED	1 TBSP	11	100
BUTTER, UNSALTED	1/2 CUP	92	810
CABBAGE, CHINESE, PAK-CHOI, CKD	1 CUP	0	20
CABBAGE, CHINESE, PE-TSAI, RAW	1 CUP	0	10
CABBAGE, COMMON, COOKED, DRNED	1 CUP	0	30
CABBAGE, COMMON, RAW	1 CUP	0	15
CABBAGE, RED, RAW	1 CUP	0	20
CABBAGE, SAVOY, RAW	1 CUP	0	20
CAKE OR PASTRY FLOUR, SIFTED	1 CUP	1	350
CAMEMBERT CHEESE	1 WEDGE	9	115
CANTALOUP, RAW	1/2 MELN	1	95
CAP'N CRUNCH CEREAL	1 OZ	3	120
CARAMELS, PLAIN OR CHOCOLATE	1 OZ	3	115
CAROB FLOUR	1 CUP	0	255
CARROT CAKE, CREMCHESE FRST, REC	1 CAKE	328	6175
CARROT CAKE, CREMCHESE FRST, REC	1 PIECE	21	385
CARROTS, CANNED, DRN, W/ SALT	1 CUP	0	35
CARROTS, CANNED, DRND, W/O SALT	1 CUP	0	35

Description of food		Fat (grams)	Food Energy (calories)
CARROTS, COOKED FROM FROZEN	1 CUP	0	55
CARROTS, COOKED FROM RAW	1 CUP	0	70
CARROTS, RAW, GRATED	1 CUP	0	45
CARROTS, RAW, WHOLE	1 CARROT	0	30
CASHEW NUTS, DRY ROASTD,SALTED	1 OZ	13	165
CASHEW NUTS, DRY ROASTD,UNSALT	1 CUP	63	785
CASHEW NUTS, DRY ROASTD,UNSALT	1 OZ	13	165
CASHEW NUTS, DRY ROASTED,SALTD	1 CUP	63	785
CASHEW NUTS, OIL ROASTD,SALTED	1 CUP	63	750
CASHEW NUTS, OIL ROASTD,SALTED	1 OZ	14	165
CASHEW NUTS, OIL ROASTD,UNSALT	1 CUP	63	750
CASHEW NUTS, OIL ROASTD,UNSALT	1 OZ	14	165
CATSUP	1 CUP	1	290
CATSUP	1 TBSP	0	15
CAULIFLOWER, COOKED FROM FROZN	1 CUP	0	35
CAULIFLOWER, COOKED FROM RAW	1 CUP	0	30
CAULIFLOWER, RAW	1 CUP	0	25
CELERY SEED	1 TSP	1	10
CELERY, PASCAL TYPE, RAW,PIECE	1 CUP	0	20
CELERY, PASCAL TYPE, RAW,STALK	1 STALK	0	5
CHEDDAR CHEESE	1 CU IN	6	70
CHEDDAR CHEESE	1 OZ	9	115
CHEDDDAR CHEESE, SHREDDED	1 CUP	37	455
CHEERIOS CEREAL	1 OZ	2	110
CHEESE CRACKERS, PLAIN	10 CRACK	3	50
CHEESE CRACKERS, SANDWCH,PEANT	1 SANDWH	2	40
CHEESE SAUCE W/ MILK, FRM MIX	1 CUP	17	305
CHEESEBURGER, 4OZ PATTY	1 SANDWH	31	525
CHEESEBURGER, REGULAR	1 SANDWH	15	300
CHEESECAKE	1 CAKE	213	3350
CHEESECAKE	1 PIECE	18	280
CHERRIES, SOUR,RED,CANND,WATER	1 CUP	0	90
CHERRIES, SWEET, RAW	10 CHERY	1	50
CHERRY PIE	1 PIE	107	2465
CHERRY PIE	1 PIECE	18	410
CHESTNUTS, EUROPEAN, ROASTED	1 CUP	3	350
CHICKEN A LA KING, HOME RECIPE	1 CUP	34	470

Description of food			Fat (grams)	Food Energy (calories)
CHICKEN AND NOODLES, HOME RECP	1 CUP		18	365
CHICKEN CHOW MEIN, CANNED	1 CUP		0	95
CHICKEN CHOW MEIN, HOME RECIPE	1 CUP		10	255
CHICKEN FRANKFURTER	1 FRANK		9	115
CHICKEN GRAVY FROM DRY MIX	1 CUP		2	85
CHICKEN GRAVY, CANNED	1 CUP		14	190
CHICKEN LIVER, COOKED	1 LIVER		1	30
CHICKEN NOODLE SOUP, CANNED	1 CUP		2	75
CHICKEN NOODLE SOUP, DEHYD, PRPD	1 PKT		1	40
CHICKEN POTPIE, HOME RECIPE	1 PIECE		31	545
CHICKEN RICE SOUP, CANNED	1 CUP		2	60
CHICKEN ROLL, LIGHT	2 SLICES		4	90
CHICKEN, CANNED, BONELESS	5 OZ		11	235
CHICKEN, FRIED, BATTER, BREAST	4.9 OZ		18	365
CHICKEN, FRIED, BATTER, DRMSTCK	2.5 OZ		11	195
CHICKEN, FRIED, FLOUR, BREAST	3.5 OZ		9	220
CHICKEN, FRIED, FLOUR, DRMSTCK	1.7 OZ		7	120
CHICKEN, ROASTED, BREAST	3.0 OZ		3	140
CHICKEN, ROASTED, DRUMSTICK	1.6 OZ		2	75
CHICKEN, STEWED, LIGHT + DARK	1 CUP		9	250
CHICKPEAS, COOKED, DRAINED	1 CUP		4	270
CHILI CON CARNE W/ BEANS, CNND	1 CUP		16	340
CHILI POWDER	1 TSP		0	10
CHOCOLATE CHIP COOKIES, COMMRCL	4 COOKIE		9	180
CHOCOLATE CHIP COOKIES, HME RCP	4 COOKIE		11	185
CHOCOLATE CHIP COOKIES, REFRIG	4 COOKIE		11	225
CHOCOLATE MILK, LOWFAT 1%	1 CUP		3	160
CHOCOLATE MILK, LOWFAT 2%	1 CUP		5	180
CHOCOLATE MILK, REGULAR	1 CUP		8	210
CHOCOLATE, BITTER OT BAKING	1 OZ		15	145
CHOP SUEY W/ BEEF + PORK, HMRCP	1 CUP		17	300
CINNAMON	1 TSP		0	5
CLAM CHOWDER, MANHATTAN, CANND	1 CUP		2	80
CLAM CHOWDER, NEW ENG, W/ MILK	1 CUP		7	165
CLAMS, CANNED, DRAINED	3 OZ		2	85
CLAMS, RAW	3 OZ		1	65
CLUB SODA	12 FL OZ		0	0

Description of food		Fat (grams)	Food Energy (calories)
COCA PWDR W/O NOFAT DRYMLK,PRD	1 SERVNG	9	225
COCA PWDR W/O NONFAT DRY MILK	3/4 OZ	1	75
COCOA PWDR WITH NONFAT DRYMILK	1 OZ	1	100
COCOA PWDR W/ NOFAT DRMLK,PRPD	1 SERVNG	1	100
COCONUT, DRIED, SWEETND,SHREDD	1 CUP	33	470
COCONUT, RAW, PIECE	1 PIECE	15	160
COCONUT, RAW, SHREDDED	1 CUP	27	285
COFFEECAKE, CRUMB, FROM MIX	1 CAKE	41	1385
COFFEECAKE, CRUMB, FROM MIX	1 PIECE	7	230
COFFEE, BREWED	6 FL OZ	0	0
COFFEE, INSTANT, PREPARED	6 FL OZ	0	0
COLA, DIET, ASPARTAME ONLY	12 FL OZ	0	0
COLA, DIET, ASPRTAME + SACCHRN	12 FL OZ	0	0
COLA, DIET, SACCHARIN ONLY	12 FL OZ	0	0
COLA, REGULAR	12 FL OZ	0	160
COLLARDS, COOKED FROM FROZEN	1 CUP	1	60
COLLARDS, COOKED FROM RAW	1 CUP	0	25
COOKED SALAD DRSSING, HOME RCP	1 TBSP	2	25
CORN CHIPS	1 OZ	9	155
CORN FLAKES, KELLOGG'S	1 OZ	0	110
CORN FLAKES, TOASTIES	1 OZ	0	110
CORN GRITS, COOKED, INSTANT	1 PKT	0	80
CORN GRITS,CKD,REG,WHTE,NOSALT	1 CUP	0	145
CORN GRITS,CKD,REG,WHTE,W/SALT	1 CUP	0	145
CORN GRITS,CKD,REG,YLLW,NOSALT	1 CUP	0	145
CORN GRITS,CKD,REG,YLLW,W/SALT	1 CUP	0	145
CORN MUFFINS, FROM COMMERL MIX	1 MUFFIN	6	145
CORN MUFFINS, HOME RECIPE	1 MUFFIN	5	145
CORN OIL	1 CUP	218	1925
CORN OIL	1 TBSP	14	125
CORNMEAL,BOLTED,DRY FORM	1 CUP	4	440
CORNMEAL,DEGERMED,ENRCHED,COOK	1 CUP	0	120
CORNMEAL,DEGERMED,ENRICHED,DRY	1 CUP	2	500
CORNMEAL,WHOLE-GRND,UNBOLT,DRY	1 CUP	5	435
CORN, CNND,CRM STL,WHIT,NO SAL	1 CUP	1	185
CORN, CNND,CRM STL,WHIT,W/SALT	1 CUP	1	185
CORN, CNND,CRM STL,YLLW,NO SAL	1 CUP	1	185

Description of food		Fat (grams)	Food Energy (calories)
CORN, CNND,CRM STL,YLLW,W/SALT	1 CUP	1	185
CORN, COOKED FRM FROZN, WHITE	1 CUP	0	135
CORN, COOKED FRM FROZN, WHITE	1 EAR	0	60
CORN, COOKED FRM FROZN, YELLOW	1 CUP	0	135
CORN, COOKED FRM FROZN, YELLOW	1 EAR	0	60
CORN, COOKED FROM RAW, WHITE	1 EAR	1	85
CORN, COOKED FROM RAW, YELLOW	1 EAR	1	85
CORN,CNND,WHL KRNL,WHTE,NO SAL	1 CUP	1	165
CORN,CNND,WHL KRNL,WHTE,W/SALT	1 CUP	1	165
CORN,CNND,WHL KRNL,YLLW,NO SAL	1 CUP	1	165
CORN,CNND,WHL KRNL,YLLW,W/SALT	1 CUP	1	165
COTTAGE CHEESE,CREMD,LRGE CURD	1 CUP	10	235
COTTAGE CHEESE,CREMD,SMLL CURD	1 CUP	9	215
COTTAGE CHEESE,CREMD,W/FRUIT	1 CUP	8	280
COTTAGE CHEESE,LOWFAT 2%	1 CUP	4	205
COTTAGE CHEESE,UNCREAMED	1 CUP	1	125
CR OF CHICKEN SOUP W/ H2O,CNND	1 CUP	7	115
CR OF CHICKEN SOUP W/ MLK,CNND	1 CUP	11	190
CR OF MUSHROM SOUP W/ H2O,CNND	1 CUP	9	130
CR OF MUSHROM SOUP W/ MLK,CNND	1 CUP	14	205
CRABMEAT, CANNED	1 CUP	3	135
CRACKED-WHEAT BREAD	1 LOAF	16	1190
CRACKED-WHEAT BREAD	1 SLICE	1	65
CRACKED-WHEAT BREAD, TOASTED	1 SLICE	1	65
CRANBERRY JUICE COCKTAL W/VITC	1 CUP	0	145
CRANBERRY SAUCE, CANNED,SWTND	1 CUP	0	420
CREAM CHEESE	1 OZ	10	100
CREAM OF WHEAT,CKD,MIX N EAT	1 PKT	0	100
CREME PIE	1 PIE	139	2710
CREME PIE	1 PIECE	23	455
CRM WHEAT,CKD, QUICK, NO SALT	1 CUP	0	140
CRM WHEAT,CKD,QUICK, W/ SALT	1 CUP	0	140
CRM WHEAT,CKD,REG,INST,NO SALT	1 CUP	0	140
CRM WHEAT,CKD,REG,INST,W/SALT	1 CUP	0	140
CROISSANTS	1 CROSST	12	235
CUCUMBER, W/ PEEL	6 SLICES	0	5
CURRY POWDER	1 TSP	0	5

Description of food		Fat (grams)	Food Energy (calories)
CUSTARD PIE	1 PIE	101	1985
CUSTARD PIE	1 PIECE	17	330
CUSTARD, BAKED	1 CUP	15	305
DANDELION GREENS, COOKED, DRND	1 CUP	1	35
DANISH PASTRY, FRUIT	1 PASTRY	13	235
DANISH PASTRY, PLAIN, NO NUTS	1 OZ	6	110
DANISH PASTRY, PLAIN, NO NUTS	1 PASTRY	12	220
DANISH PASTRY, PLAIN, NO NUTS	1 RING	71	1305
DATES	10 DATES	0	230
DATES, CHOPPED	1 CUP	1	490
DEVIL'S FOOD CAKE,CHOCFRST,FMX	1 CAKE	136	3755
DEVIL'S FOOD CAKE,CHOCFRST,FMX	1 CUPCAK	4	120
DEVIL'S FOOD CAKE,CHOCFRST,FMX	1 PIECE	8	235
DOUGHNUTS, CAKE TYPE, PLAIN	1 DONUT	12	210
DOUGHNUTS, YEAST-LEAVEND,GLZED	1 DONUT	13	235
DUCK, ROASTED, FLESH ONLY	1/2 DUCK	25	445
EGGNOG	1 CUP	19	340
EGGPLANT, COOKED, STEAMED	1 CUP	0	25
EGGS, COOKED, FRIED	1 EGG	7	90
EGGS, COOKED, HARD-COOKED	1 EGG	5	75
EGGS, COOKED, POACHED	1 EGG	5	75
EGGS, COOKED, SCRAMBLED/OMELET	1 EGG	7	100
EGGS, RAW, WHITE	1 WHITE	0	15
EGGS, RAW, WHOLE	1 EGG	5	75
EGGS, RAW, YOLK	1 YOLK	5	60
ENCHILADA	1 ENCHLD	16	235
ENDIVE, CURLY, RAW	1 CUP	0	10
ENG MUFFIN, EGG, CHEESE, BACON	1 SANDWH	18	360
ENGLISH MUFFINS, PLAIN	1 MUFFIN	1	140
ENGLISH MUFFINS, PLAIN, TOASTD	1 MUFFIN	1	140
EVAPORATED MILK, SKIM, CANNED	1 CUP	1	200
EVAPORATED MILK, WHOLE, CANNED	1 CUP	19	340
FATS, COOKING/VEGETBL SHORTENG	1 CUP	205	1810
FATS, COOKING/VEGETBL SHORTENG	1 TBSP	13	115
FETA CHEESE	1 OZ	6	75
FIG BARS	4 COOKIE	4	210
FIGS, DRIED	10 FIGS	2	475

Description of food		Fat (grams)	Food Energy (calories)
FILBERTS, (HAZELNUTS) CHOPPED	1 CUP	72	725
FILBERTS, (HAZELNUTS) CHOPPED	1 OZ	18	180
FISH SANDWICH, LGE, W/O CHEESE	1 SANDWH	27	470
FISH SANDWICH, REG, W/ CHEESE	1 SANDWH	23	420
FISH STICKS, FROZEN, REHEATED	1 STICK	3	70
FLOUNDER OR SOLE, BAKED, BUTTR	3 OZ	6	120
FLOUNDER OR SOLE, BAKED, MARGRN	3 OZ	6	120
FLOUNDER OR SOLE, BAKED, W/OFAT	3 OZ	1	80
FONDANT, UNCOATED	1 OZ	0	105
FRANKFURTER, COOKED	1 FRANK	13	145
FRENCH BREAD	1 SLICE	1	100
FRENCH OR VIENNA BREAD	1 LOAF	18	1270
FRENCH SALAD DRESSING, LOCALOR	1 TBSP	2	25
FRENCH SALAD DRESSING, REGULAR	1 TBSP	9	85
FRENCH TOAST, HOME RECIPE	1 SLICE	7	155
FRIED PIE, APPLE	1 PIE	14	255
FRIED PIE, CHERRY	1 PIE	14	250
FROOT LOOPS CEREAL	1 OZ	1	110
FRUIT COCKTAIL, CNND, HEAVYSYRUP	1 CUP	0	185
FRUIT COCKTAIL, CNND, JUICE PACK	1 CUP	0	115
FRUIT PUNCH DRINK, CANNED	6 FL OZ	0	85
FRUITCAKE, DARK, FROM HOMERECIP	1 CAKE	228	5185
FRUITCAKE, DARK, FROM HOMERECIP	1 PIECE	7	165
FUDGE, CHOCOLATE, PLAIN	1 OZ	3	115
GARLIC POWDER	1 TSP	0	10
GELATIN DESSERT, PREPARED	1/2 CUP	0	70
GELATIN, DRY	1 ENVELP	0	25
GINGER ALE	12 FL OZ	0	125
GINGERBREAD CAKE, FROM MIX	1 CAKE	39	1575
GINGERBREAD CAKE, FROM MIX	1 PIECE	4	175
GIN, RUM, VODKA, WHISKY 80-PROOF	1.5 F OZ	0	95
GIN, RUM, VODKA, WHISKY 86-PROOF	1.5 F OZ	0	105
GIN, RUM, VODKA, WHISKY 90-PROOF	1.5 F OZ	0	110
GOLDEN GRAHAMS CEREAL	1 OZ	1	110
GRAHAM CRACKER, PLAIN	2 CRACKR	1	60
GRAPE-NUTS CEREAL	1 OZ	0	100
GRAPE DRINK, CANNED	6 FL OZ	0	100

Description of food		Fat (grams)	Food Energy (calories)
GRAPE JUICE, CANNED	1 CUP	0	155
GRAPE SODA	12 FL OZ	0	180
GRAPEFRT JCE,FRZN,CNCN,UNSWTEN	6 FL OZ	1	300
GRAPEFRT JCE,FRZN,DLTD,UNSWTEN	1 CUP	0	100
GRAPEFRUIT JUICE, CANNED,SWTND	1 CUP	0	115
GRAPEFRUIT JUICE, CANNED,UNSWT	1 CUP	0	95
GRAPEFRUIT JUICE, RAW	1 CUP	0	95
GRAPEFRUIT, CANNED, SYRUP PACK	1 CUP	0	150
GRAPEFRUIT, RAW, PINK	1/2 FRUT	0	40
GRAPEFRUIT, RAW, WHITE	1/2 FRUT	0	40
GRAPEJCE,FRZN,CONCEN,SWTND,W/C	6 FL OZ	1	385
GRAPEJCE,FRZN,DILUTD,SWTND,W/C	1 CUP	0	125
GRAPES, EUROPEAN, RAW, THOMPSN	10 GRAPE	0	35
GRAPES, EUROPEAN, RAW, TOKAY	10 GRAPE	0	40
GRAVY AND TURKEY, FROZEN	5 OZ	4	95
GREAT NORTHN BEANS,DRY,CKD,DRN	1 CUP	1	210
GROUND BEEF, BROILED, LEAN	3 OZ	16	230
GROUND BEEF, BROILED, REGULAR	3 OZ	18	245
GUM DROPS	1 OZ	0	100
HADDOCK, BREADED, FRIED	3 OZ	9	175
HALF AND HALF, CREAM	1 CUP	28	315
HALF AND HALF, CREAM	1 TBSP	2	20
HALIBUT, BROILED, BUTTER,LEMJU	3 OZ	6	140
HAMBURGER, 4OZ PATTY	1 SANDWH	21	445
HAMBURGER, REGULAR	1 SANDWH	11	245
HARD CANDY	1 OZ	0	110
HERRING, PICKLED	3 OZ	13	190
HOLLANDAISE SCE, W/ H2O,FRM MX	1 CUP	20	240
HONEY	1 CUP	0	1030
HONEY	1 TBSP	0	65
HONEY NUT CHEERIOS CEREAL	1 OZ	1	105
HONEYDEW MELON, RAW	1/10 MEL	0	45
ICE CREAM, VANLLA, REGULR 11%	1 CUP	14	270
ICE CREAM, VANLLA, REGULR 11%	1/2 GALN	115	2155
ICE CREAM, VANLLA, REGULR 11%	3 FL OZ	5	100
ICE CREAM, VANLLA, RICH 16% FT	1 CUP	24	350
ICE CREAM, VANLLA, RICH 16% FT	1/2 GAL	190	2805

Description of food			Fat (grams)	Food Energy (calories)
ICE CREAM, VANLLA, SOFT SERVE	1 CUP		23	375
ICE MILK, VANILLA, 4% FAT	1 CUP		6	185
ICE MILK, VANILLA, 4% FAT	1/2 GAL		45	1470
ICE MILK, VANILLA, SOFTSERV 3%	1 CUP		5	225
IMITATION CREAMERS, LIQUID FRZ	1 TBSP		1	20
IMITATION CREAMERS, POWDERED	1 TSP		1	10
IMITATION WHIPPED TOPPING, FRZN	1 CUP		19	240
IMITATION WHIPPED TOPPING, FRZN	1 TBSP		1	15
IMITATN SOUR DRESSING	1 CUP		39	415
IMITATN SOUR DRESSING	1 TBSP		2	20
IMITATN WHIPD TOPING, PRESSRZD	1 CUP		16	185
IMITATN WHIPD TOPING, PRESSRZD	1 TBSP		1	10
IMITATN WHIPD TOPING, PWDRD, PRP	1 CUP		10	150
IMITATN WHIPD TOPING, PWDRD, PRP	1 TBSP		0	10
ITALIAN BREAD	1 LOAF		4	1255
ITALIAN BREAD	1 SLICE		0	85
ITALIAN SALAD DRESSING, LOCALOR	1 TBSP		0	5
ITALIAN SALAD DRESSING, REGULAR	1 TBSP		9	80
JAMS AND PRESERVES	1 PKT		0	40
JAMS AND PRESERVES	1 TBSP		0	55
JELLIES	1 PKT		0	40
JELLIES	1 TBSP		0	50
JELLY BEANS	1 OZ		0	105
JERUSALEM-ARTICHOKE, RAW	1 CUP		0	115
KALE, COOKED FROM FROZEN	1 CUP		1	40
KALE, COOKED FROM RAW	1 CUP		1	40
KIWIFRUIT, RAW	1 KIWI		0	45
KOHLRABI, COOKED, DRAINED	1 CUP		0	50
LAMB, RIB, ROASTED, LEAN ONLY	2 OZ		7	130
LAMB, RIB, ROASTED, LEAN + FAT	3 OZ		26	315
LAMB, CHOPS, ARM, BRAISED, LEAN	1.7 OZ		7	135
LAMB, CHOPS, ARM, BRAISED, LEAN+FT	2.2 OZ		15	220
LAMB, CHOPS, LOIN, BROIL, LEAN	2.3 OZ		6	140
LAMB, CHOPS, LOIN, BROIL, LEAN+FAT	2.8 OZ		16	235
LAMB, LEG, ROASTED, LEAN ONLY	2.6 OZ		6	140
LAMB, LEG, ROASTED, LEAN+ FAT	3 OZ		13	205
LARD	1 CUP		205	1850

Description of food		Fat (grams)	Food Energy (calories)
LARD	1 TBSP	13	115
LEMON-LIME SODA	12 FL OZ	0	155
LEMON JUICE, CANNED	1 CUP	1	50
LEMON JUICE, CANNED	1 TBSP	0	5
LEMON JUICE, RAW	1 CUP	0	60
LEMON JUICE,FRZN,SINGLE-STRNGH	6 FL OZ	1	55
LEMON MERINGUE PIE	1 PIE	86	2140
LEMON MERINGUE PIE	1 PIECE	14	355
LEMONADE,CONCENTRATE,FRZ,UNDIL	6 FL OZ	0	425
LEMONADE,CONCEN,FRZEN,DILUTED	6 FL OZ	0	80
LEMONS, RAW	1 LEMON	0	15
LENTILS, DRY, COOKED	1 CUP	1	215
LETTUCE, BUTTERHEAD, RAW,HEAD	1 HEAD	0	20
LETTUCE, BUTTERHEAD, RAW,LEAVE	1 LEAF	0	0
LETTUCE, CRISPHEAD, RAW, HEAD	1 HEAD	1	70
LETTUCE, CRISPHEAD, RAW,PIECES	1 CUP	0	5
LETTUCE, CRISPHEAD, RAW,WEDGE	1 WEDGE	0	20
LETTUCE, LOOSELEAF	1 CUP	0	10
LIGHT, COFFEE OR TABLE CREAM	1 CUP	46	470
LIGHT, COFFEE OR TABLE CREAM	1 TBSP	3	30
LIMA BEANS, DRY, COOKED,DRANED	1 CUP	1	260
LIMA BEANS,BABY, FRZN,CKED,DRN	1 CUP	1	190
LIMA BEANS,THICK SEED,FRZN,CKD	1 CUP	1	170
LIME JUICE, RAW	1 CUP	0	65
LIME JUICE,CANNED	1 CUP	1	50
LIMEADE,CONCENTRATE,FRZN,UNDIL	6 FL OZ	0	410
LIMEADE,CONCEN,FROZEN,DILUTED	6 FL OZ	0	75
LUCKY CHARMS CEREAL	1 OZ	1	110
MACADAMIA NUTS, OILRSTD,SALTED	1 CUP	103	960
MACADAMIA NUTS, OILRSTD,SALTED	1 OZ	22	205
MACADAMIA NUTS, OILRSTD,UNSALT	1 CUP	103	960
MACADAMIA NUTS, OILRSTD,UNSALT	1 OZ	22	205
MACARONI AND CHEESE, CANNED	1 CUP	10	230
MACARONI AND CHEESE, HOME RCPE	1 CUP	22	430
MACARONI, COOKED, FIRM	1 CUP	1	190
MACARONI, COOKED, TENDER, HOT	1 CUP	1	155
MACARONI, COOKED, TENDER,COLD	1 CUP	0	115

Description of food		Fat (grams)	Food Energy (calories)
MALT-O-MEAL, WITH SALT	1 CUP	0	120
MALT-O-MEAL, W/O SALT	1 CUP	0	120
MALTED MILK, CHOCOLATE, POWDER	3/4 OZ	1	85
MALTED MILK, CHOCOLATE, PWDRPPD	1 SERVNG	9	235
MALTED MILK, NATURAL, POWDER	3/4 OZ	2	85
MALTED MILK, NATURAL, PWDR PPRD	1 SERVNG	10	235
MANGOS, RAW	1 MANGO	1	135
MARGARINE, IMITATION 40% FAT	1 TBSP	5	50
MARGARINE, IMITATION 40% FAT	8 OZ	88	785
MARGARINE, REGULR, HARD, 80% FAT	1 PAT	4	35
MARGARINE, REGULR, HARD, 80% FAT	1 TBSP	11	100
MARGARINE, REGULR, HARD, 80% FAT	1/2 CUP	91	810
MARGARINE, REGULR, SOFT, 80% FAT	1 TBSP	11	100
MARGARINE, REGULR, SOFT, 80% FAT	8 OZ	183	1625
MARGARINE, SPREAD, HARD, 60% FAT	1 PAT	3	25
MARGARINE, SPREAD, HARD, 60% FAT	1 TBSP	9	75
MARGARINE, SPREAD, HARD, 60% FAT	1/2 CUP	69	610
MARGARINE, SPREAD, SOFT, 60% FAT	1 TBSP	9	75
MARGARINE, SPREAD, SOFT, 60% FAT	8 OZ	138	1225
MARSHMALLOWS	1 OZ	0	90
MAYONNAISE TYPE SALAD DRESSING	1 TBSP	5	60
MAYONNAISE, IMITATION	1 TBSP	3	35
MAYONNAISE, REGULAR	1 TBSP	11	100
MELBA TOAST, PLAIN	1 PIECE	0	20
MILK CHOCOLATE CANDY, PLAIN	1 OZ	9	145
MILK CHOCOLATE CANDY, W/ ALMOND	1 OZ	10	150
MILK CHOCOLATE CANDY, W/ PENUTS	1 OZ	11	155
MILK CHOCOLATE CANDY, W/ RICE C	1 OZ	7	140 ·
MILK, LOFAT, 1%, ADDED SOLIDS	1 CUP	2	105
MILK, LOFAT, 1%, NO ADDEDSOLID	1 CUP	3	100
MILK, LOFAT, 2%, ADDED SOLIDS	1 CUP	5	125
MILK, LOFAT, 2%, NO ADDEDSOLID	1 CUP	5	120
MILK, SKIM, ADDED MILK SOLIDS	1 CUP	1	90
MILK, SKIM, NO ADDED MILKSOLID	1 CUP	0	85
MILK, WHOLE, 3.3% FAT	1 CUP	8	150
MINESTRONE SOUP, CANNED	1 CUP	3	80
MISO	1 CUP	13	470

Description of food			Fat (grams)	Food Energy (calories)
MIXED GRAIN BREAD	1	LOAF	17	1165
MIXED GRAIN BREAD	1	SLICE	1	65
MIXED GRAIN BREAD, TOASTED	1	SLICE	1	65
MIXED NUTS W/ PEANTS,DRY,SALTD	1	OZ	15	170
MIXED NUTS W/ PEANTS,DRY,UNSLT	1	OZ	15	170
MIXED NUTS W/ PEANTS,OIL,SALTD	1	OZ	16	175
MIXED NUTS W/ PEANTS,OIL,UNSLT	1	OZ	16	175
MOLASSES, CANE, BLACKSTRAP	2	TBSP	0	85
MOZZARELLA CHEESE, WHOLE MILK	1	OZ	6	80
MOZZARELLA CHESE,SKIM, LOMOIST	1	OZ	5	80
MUENSTER CHEESE	1	OZ	9	105
MUSHROOM GRAVY, CANNED	1	CUP	6	120
MUSHROOMS, CANNED, DRND,W/SALT	1	CUP	0	35
MUSHROOMS, COOKED, DRAINED	1	CUP	1	40
MUSHROOMS, RAW	1	CUP	0	20
MUSTARD GREENS, COOKED, DRANED	1	CUP	0	20
MUSTARD, PREPARED, YELLOW	1	TSP	0	5
NATURE VALLEY GRANOLA CEREAL	1	OZ	5	125
NECTARINES, RAW	1	NECTRN	1	65
NONFAT DRY MILK, INSTANTIZED	1	CUP	0	245
NONFAT DRY MILK, INSTANTIZED	1	ENVLPE	1	325
NOODLES, CHOW MEIN, CANNED	1	CUP	11	220
NOODLES, EGG, COOKED	1	CUP	2	200
OATMEAL BREAD	1	LOAF	20	1145
OATMEAL BREAD	1	SLICE	1	65
OATMEAL BREAD, TOASTED	1	SLICE	1	65
OATMEAL W/ RAISINS COOKIES	4	COOKIE	10	245
OATMEAL,CKD,INSTNT,FLVRD,FORTF	1	PKT	2	160
OATMEAL,CKD,INSTNT,PLAIN,FORTF	1	PKT	2	105
OATMEAL,CKD,RG,QCK,INST,W/OSAL	1	CUP	2	145
OATMEAL,CKD,RG,QCK,INST,W/SALT	1	CUP	2	145
OCEAN PERCH, BREADED, FRIED	1	FILLET	11	185
OKRA PODS, COOKED	8	PODS	0	25
OLIVE OIL	1	CUP	216	1910
OLIVE OIL	1	TBSP	14	125
OLIVES, CANNED, GREEN	4	MEDIUM	2	15
OLIVES, CANNED, RIPE, MISSION	3	SMALL	2	15

Description of food		Fat (grams)	Food Energy (calories)
ONION POWDER	1 TSP	0	5
ONION RINGS, BREADED,FRZN,PRPD	2 RINGS	5	80
ONION SOUP, DEHYDRATD, PREPRED	1 PKT	0	20
ONION SOUP, DEHYDRTD, UNPRPRED	1 PKT	0	20
ONIONS, RAW, CHOPPED	1 CUP	0	55
ONIONS, RAW, COOKED, DRAINED	1 CUP	0	60
ONIONS, RAW, SLICED	1 CUP	0	40
ONIONS, SPRING, RAW	6 ONION	0	10
ORANGE JUICE, CANNED	1 CUP	0	105
ORANGE JUICE, CHILLED	1 CUP	1	110
ORANGE JUICE, RAW	1 CUP	0	110
ORANGE JUICE,FROZEN CONCENTRTE	6 FL OZ	0	340
ORANGE JUICE,FRZN,CNCN,DILUTED	1 CUP	0	110
ORANGE SODA	12 FL OZ	0	180
ORANGE + GRAPEFRUIT JUCE,CANND	1 CUP	0	105
ORANGES, RAW	1 ORANGE	0	60
ORANGES, RAW, SECTIONS	1 CUP	0	85
OREGANO	1 TSP	0	5
OYSTERS, BREADED, FRIED	1 OYSTER	5	90
OYSTERS, RAW	1 CUP	4	160
PANCAKES, BUCKWHEAT, FROM MIX	1 PANCAK	2	55
PANCAKES, PLAIN, FROM MIX	1 PANCAK	2	60
PANCAKES, PLAIN, HOME RECIPE	1 PANCAK	2	60
PAPRIKA	1 TSP	0	5
PARMESAN CHEESE, GRATED	1 CUP	30	455
PARMESAN CHEESE, GRATED	1 OZ	9	130
PARMESAN CHEESE, GRATED	1 TBSP	2	25
PARSLEY, FREEZE-DRIED	1 TBSP	0	0
PARSLEY, RAW	10 SPRIG	0	5
PARSNIPS, COOKED, DRAINED	1 CUP	0	125
PASTERZD PROCES CHEESE, SWISS	1 OZ	7	95
PASTERZD PROCES CHEESE,AMERICN	1 OZ	9	105
PASTERZD PROCES CHESE FOOD,AMR	1 OZ	7	95
PASTERZD PROCES CHESE SPRED,AM	1 OZ	6	80
PEA BEANS, DRY, COOKED,DRAINED	1 CUP	1	225
PEACH PIE	1 PIE	101	2410
PEACH PIE	1 PIECE	17	405
PEACHES, CANNED, HEAVY SYRUP	1 CUP	0	190

Description of food			Fat (grams)	Food Energy (calories)
PEACHES, CANNED, HEAVY SYRUP	1	HALF	0	60
PEACHES, CANNED, JUICE PACK	1	CUP	0	110
PEACHES, CANNED, JUICE PACK	1	HALF	0	35
PEACHES, DRIED	1	CUP	1	380
PEACHES, DRIED,COOKED,UNSWETND	1	CUP	1	200
PEACHES, FROZEN,SWETNED,W/VITC	1	CUP	0	235
PEACHES, FROZEN,SWETNED,W/VITC	10	OZ	0	265
PEACHES, RAW	1	PEACH	0	35
PEACHES, RAW, SLICED	1	CUP	0	75
PEANUT BUTTER	1	TBSP	8	95
PEANUT BUTTER COOKIE,HOME RECP	4	COOKIE	14	245
PEANUT OIL	1	CUP	216	1910
PEANUT OIL	1	TBSP	14	125
PEANUTS, OIL ROASTED, SALTED	1	CUP	71	840
PEANUTS, OIL ROASTED, SALTED	1	OZ	14	165
PEANUTS, OIL ROASTED, UNSALTED	1	CUP	71	840
PEANUTS, OIL ROASTED, UNSALTED	1	OZ	14	165
PEARS, CANNED, HEAVY SYRUP	1	CUP	0	190
PEARS, CANNED, HEAVY SYRUP	1	HALF	0	60
PEARS, CANNED, JUICE PACK	1	CUP	0	125
PEARS, CANNED, JUICE PACK	1	HALF	0	40
PEARS, RAW, BARTLETT	1	PEAR	1	100
PEARS, RAW, BOSC	1	PEAR	1	85
PEARS, RAW, D'ANJOU	1	PEAR	1	120
PEAS, EDIBLE POD, COOKED,DRNED	1	CUP	0	65
PEAS, GREEN,CNND,DRND, W/ SALT	1	CUP	1	115
PEAS, GREEN,CNND,DRND,W/O SALT	1	CUP	1	115
PEAS, SPLIT, DRY, COOKED	1	CUP	1	230
PEAS,GRN, FROZEN COOKED,DRANED	1	CUP	0	125
PEA, GREEN, SOUP, CANNED	1	CUP	3	165
PECAN PIE	1	PIE	189	3450
PECAN PIE	1	PIECE	32	575
PECANS, HALVES	1	CUP	73	720
PECANS, HALVES	1	OZ	19	190
PEPPER-TYPE SODA	12	FL OZ	0	160
PEPPERS, HOT CHILI, RAW, GREEN	1	PEPPER	0	20
PEPPERS, HOT CHILI, RAW, RED	1	PEPPER	0	20

Description of food		Fat (grams)	Food Energy (calories)
PEPPERS, SWEET, COOKED, GREEN	1 PEPPER	0	15
PEPPERS, SWEET, COOKED, RED	1 PEPPER	0	15
PEPPERS, SWEET, RAW, GREEN	1 PEPPER	0	20
PEPPERS, SWEET, RAW, RED	1 PEPPER	0	20
PEPPER, BLACK	1 TSP	0	5
PICKLES, CUCUMBER, DILL	1 PICKLE	0	5
PICKLES, CUCUMBER, FRESH PACK	2 SLICES	0	10
PICKLES, CUCUMBER, SWT GHERKIN	1 PICKLE	0	20
PIECRUST, FROM MIX	2 CRUST	93	1485
PIECRUST, FROM HOME RECIPE	1 SHELL	60	900
PINE NUTS	1 OZ	17	160
PINEAPPLE-GRAPEFRUIT JUICEDRNK	6 FL OZ	0	90
PINEAPPLE JUICE, CANNED,UNSWTN	1 CUP	0	140
PINEAPPLE, CANNED, HEAVY SYRUP	1 CUP	0	200
PINEAPPLE, CANNED, HEAVY SYRUP	1 SLICE	0	45
PINEAPPLE, CANNED, JUICE PACK	1 CUP	0	150
PINEAPPLE, CANNED, JUICE PACK	1 SLICE	0	35
PINEAPPLE, RAW, DICED	1 CUP	1	75
PINTO BEANS,DRY,COOKED,DRAINED	1 CUP	1	265
PISTACHIO NUTS	1 OZ	14	165
PITA BREAD	1 PITA	1	165
PIZZA, CHEESE	1 SLICE	9	290
PLANTAINS, COOKED	1 CUP	0	180
PLANTAINS, RAW	1 PLANTN	1	220
PLUMS, CANNED, HEAVY SYRUP	1 CUP	0	230
PLUMS, CANNED, HEAVY SYRUP	3 PLUMS	0	120
PLUMS, CANNED, JUICE PACK	1 CUP	0	145
PLUMS, CANNED, JUICE PACK	3 PLUMS	0	55
PLUMS, RAW, 1-1/2-IN DIAM	1 PLUM	0	15
PLUMS, RAW, 2-1/8-IN DIAM	1 PLUM	0	35
POPCORN, AIR-POPPED, UNSALTED	1 CUP	0	30
POPCORN, POPPED, VEG OIL,SALTD	1 CUP	3	55
POPCORN, SUGAR SYRUP COATED	1 CUP	1	135
POPSICLE	1 POPCLE	0	70
PORK CHOP, LOIN, BROIL, LEAN	2.5 OZ	8	165
PORK CHOP, LOIN, BROIL, LEN+FT	3.1 OZ	19	275
PORK CHOP, LOIN,PANFRY, LEAN	2.4 OZ	11	180

Description of food	Fat (grams)	Food Energy (calories)
PORK CHOP, LOIN,PANFRY,LEAN+FT3.1 OZ	27	335
PORK FRESH HAM, ROASTD, LEAN 2.5 OZ	8	160
PORK FRESH HAM, ROASTD,LEAN+FT3 OZ	18	250
PORK FRESH RIB, ROASTD, LEAN 2.5 OZ	10	175
PORK FRESH RIB, ROASTD,LEAN+FT3 OZ	20	270
PORK SHOULDER, BRAISD, LEAN 2.4 OZ	8	165
PORK SHOULDER, BRAISD,LEAN+FAT3 OZ	22	295
PORK, CURED, BACON, REGUL,CKED3 SLICE	9	110
PORK, CURED, BACON,CANADN,CKED2 SLICE	4	85
PORK, CURED, HAM, CANNED,ROAST3 OZ	7	140
PORK, CURED, HAM, ROSTED,LEAN 2.4 OZ	4	105
PORK, CURED, HAM, ROSTED,LN+FT3 OZ	14	205
PORK, LINK, COOKED 1 LINK	4	50
PORK, LUNCHEON MEAT,CANNED 2 SLICES	13	140
PORK, LUNCHEON MEAT,CHOPPD HAM2 SLICES	7	95
PORK, LUNCHEON MEAT,CKD HAM,LN2 SLICES	3	75
PORK, LUNCHEON MEAT,CKD HAM,RG2 SLICES	6	105
POTATO CHIPS 10 CHIPS	7	105
POTATO SALAD MADE W/ MAYONNAIS1 CUP	21	360
POTATOES, AU GRATIN, FROM MIX 1 CUP	10	230
POTATOES, AU GRATIN, HOME RECP1 CUP	19	325
POTATOES, BAKED FLESH ONLY 1 POTATO	0	145
POTATOES, BAKED WITH SKIN 1 POTATO	0	220
POTATOES, BOILED, PEELED AFTER1 POTATO	0	120
POTATOES, BOILED, PEELED BEFOR1 POTATO	0	115
POTATOES, HASHED BROWN,FR FRZN1 CUP	18	340
POTATOES, MASHED,FRM DEHYDRTED1 CUP	12	235
POTATOES, MASHED,RECPE,MLK+MAR1 CUP	9	225
POTATOES, MASHED,RECPE,W/ MILK1 CUP	1	160
POTATOES, SCALLOPED, FROM MIX 1 CUP	11	230
POTATOES, SCALLOPED, HOME RECP1 CUP	9	210
POTATOES,FRENCH-FRD,FRZN,FRIED10 STRIP	8	160
POTATOES,FRENCH-FRD,FRZN,OVEN 10 STRIP	4	110
POUND CAKE, COMMERCIAL 1 LOAF	94	1935
POUND CAKE, COMMERCIAL 1 SLICE	5	110
POUND CAKE, FROM HOME RECIPE 1 LOAF	94	2025
POUND CAKE, FROM HOME RECIPE 1 SLICE	5	120

Description of food		Fat (grams)	Food Energy (calories)
PRETZELS, STICK	10 PRETZ	0	10
PRETZELS, TWISTED, DUTCH	1 PRETZ	1	65
PRETZELS, TWISTED, THIN	10 PRETZ	2	240
PRODUCT 19 CEREAL	1 OZ	0	110
PROVOLONE CHEESE	1 OZ	8	100
PRUNE JUICE, CANNED	1 CUP	0	180
PRUNES, DRIED	5 LARGE	0	115
PRUNES, DRIED, COOKED,UNSWTNED	1 CUP	0	225
PUDDING, CHOCOLATE,CANNED	5 OZ	11	205
PUDDING, CHOC, COOKED FROM MIX	1/2 CUP	4	150
PUDDING, CHOC, INSTANT, FR MIX	1/2 CUP	4	155
PUDDING, RICE, FROM MIX	1/2 CUP	4	155
PUDDING, TAPIOCA, CANNED	5 OZ	5	160
PUDDING, TAPIOCA, FROM MIX	1/2 CUP	4	145
PUDDING, VANILLA, CANNED	5 OZ	10	220
PUDDING, VNLLA,COOKED FROM MIX	1/2 CUP	4	145
PUDDING, VNLLA,INSTANT FRM MIX	1/2 CUP	4	150
PUMPERNICKEL BREAD	1 LOAF	16	1160
PUMPERNICKEL BREAD	1 SLICE	1	80
PUMPERNICKEL BREAD, TOASTED	1 SLICE	1	80
PUMPKIN AND SQUASH KERNELS	1 OZ	13	155
PUMPKIN PIE	1 PIE	102	1920
PUMPKIN PIE	1 PIECE	17	320
PUMPKIN, CANNED	1 CUP	1	85
PUMPKIN, COOKED FROM RAW	1 CUP	0	50
QUICHE LORRAINE	1 SLICE	48	600
RADISHES, RAW	4 RADISH	0	5
RAISIN BRAN, KELLOGG'S	1 OZ	1	90
RAISIN BRAN, POST	1 OZ	1	85
RAISIN BREAD	1 LOAF	18	1260
RAISIN BREAD	1 SLICE	1	65
RAISIN BREAD, TOASTED	1 SLICE	1	65
RAISINS	1 CUP	1	435
RAISINS	1 PACKET	0	40
RASPBERRIES, FROZEN, SWEETENED	1 CUP	0	255
RASPBERRIES, FROZEN, SWEETENED	10 OZ	0	295
RASPBERRIES, RAW	1 CUP	1	60

Description of food		Fat (grams)	Food Energy (calories)
RED KIDNEY BEANS, DRY, CANNED	1 CUP	1	230
REFRIED BEANS, CANNED	1 CUP	3	295
RELISH, SWEET	1 TBSP	0	20
RHUBARB, COOKED, ADDED SUGAR	1 CUP	0	280
RICE KRISPIES CEREAL	1 OZ	0	110
RICE, BROWN, COOKED	1 CUP	1	230
RICE, WHITE, COOKED	1 CUP	0	225
RICE, WHITE, INSTANT, COOKED	1 CUP	0	180
RICE, WHITE, PARBOILED, COOKED	1 CUP	0	185
RICE, WHITE, PARBOILED, RAW	1 CUP	1	685
RICE, WHITE, RAW	1 CUP	1	670
RICOTTA CHEESE, PART SKIM MILK	1 CUP	19	340
RICOTTA CHEESE, WHOLE MILK	1 CUP	32	430
ROAST BEEF SANDWICH	1 SANDWH	13	345
ROLLS, DINNER, COMMERCIAL	1 ROLL	2	85
ROLLS, DINNER, HOME RECIPE	1 ROLL	3	120
ROLLS, FRANKFURTER + HAMBURGER	1 ROLL	2	115
ROLLS, HARD	1 ROLL	2	155
ROLLS, HOAGIE OR SUBMARINE	1 ROLL	8	400
ROOT BEER	12 FL OZ	0	165
RYE BREAD, LIGHT	1 LOAF	17	1190
RYE BREAD, LIGHT	1 SLICE	1	65
RYE BREAD, LIGHT, TOASTED	1 SLICE	1	65
RYE WAFERS, WHOLE-GRAIN	2 WAFERS	1	55
SAFFLOWER OIL	1 CUP	218	1925
SAFFLOWER OIL	1 TBSP	14	125
SALAMI, COOKED TYPE	2 SLICES	11	145
SALAMI, DRY TYPE	2 SLICES	7	85
SALMON, BAKED, RED	3 OZ	5	140
SALMON, CANNED, PINK, W/ BONES	3 OZ	5	120
SALMON, SMOKED	3 OZ	8	150
SALT	1 TSP	0	0
SALTINES	4 CRACKR	1	50
SANDWICH SPREAD, PORK, BEEF	1 TBSP	3	35
SANDWICH TYPE COOKIE	4 COOKIE	8	195
SARDINES, ATLNTC,CNNED,OIL,DRN	3 OZ	9	175
SAUERKRAUT, CANNED	1 CUP	0	45

Description of food		Fat (grams)	Food Energy (calories)
SCALLOPS, BREADED, FRZN,REHEAT	6 SCALOP	10	195
SEAWEED, KELP, RAW	1 OZ	0	10
SEAWEED, SPIRULINA, DRIED	1 OZ	2	80
SELF-RISING FLOUR, UNSIFTED	1 CUP	1	440
SEMISWEET CHOCOLATE	1 CUP	61	860
SESAME SEEDS	1 TBSP	4	45
SHAKES, THICK, CHOCOLATE	10 OZ	8	335
SHAKES, THICK, VANILLA	10 OZ	9	315
SHEETCAKE W/O FRSTNG,HOMERECIP	1 CAKE	108	2830
SHEETCAKE,W/ WHFRSTNG,HOMERCIP	1 CAKE	129	4020
SHEETCAKE,W/ WHFRSTNG,HOMERCIP	1 PIECE	14	445
SHEETCAKE,W/O FRSTNG,HOMERECIP	1 PIECE	12	315
SHERBET, 2% FAT	1 CUP	4	270
SHERBET, 2% FAT	1/2 GAL	31	2160
SHORTBREAD COOKIE, COMMERCIAL	4 COOKIE	8	155
SHORTBREAD COOKIE, HOME RECIPE	2 COOKIE	8	145
SHREDDED WHEAT CEREAL	1 OZ	1	100
SHRIMP, CANNED, DRAINED	3 OZ	1	100
SHRIMP, FRENCH FRIED	3 OZ	10	200
SNACK CAKES,DEVILS FOOD,CREMFLSM	CAKE	4	105
SNACK CAKES,SPONGE CREME FLLNGSM	CAKE	5	155
SNACK TYPE CRACKERS	1 CRACKR	1	15
SNAP BEAN,CNND,DRND,GREEN,SALT	1 CUP	0	25
SNAP BEAN,CNND,DRND,GRN,NOSALT	1 CUP	0	25
SNAP BEAN,CNND,DRND,YLLW, SALT	1 CUP	0	25
SNAP BEAN,CNND,DRND,YLLW,NOSAL	1 CUP	0	25
SNAP BEAN,FRZ,CKD,DRND,GREEN	1 CUP	0	35
SNAP BEAN,FRZ,CKD,DRND,YELLOW	1 CUP	0	35
SNAP BEAN,RAW,CKD,DRND,GREEN	1 CUP	0	45
SNAP BEAN,RAW,CKD,DRND,YELLOW	1 CUP	0	45
SOUR CREAM	1 CUP	48	495
SOUR CREAM	1 TBSP	3	25
SOY SAUCE	1 TBSP	0	10
SOYBEAN-COTTONSEED OIL, HYDRGN	1 CUP	218	1925
SOYBEAN-COTTONSEED OIL, HYDRGN	1 TBSP	14	125
SOYBEAN OIL, HYDROGENATED	1 CUP	218	1925
SOYBEAN OIL, HYDROGENATED	1 TBSP	14	125

Description of food		Fat (grams)	Food Energy (calories)
SOYBEANS, DRY, COOKED, DRAINED	1 CUP	10	235
SPAGHETTI, COOKED, FIRM	1 CUP	1	190
SPAGHETTI, COOKED, TENDER	1 CUP	1	155
SPAGHETTI, TOM SAUCE CHEES,CND	1 CUP	2	190
SPAGHETTI, TOM SAUCE CHEE,HMRP	1 CUP	9	260
SPAGHETTI,MEATBALLS,TOMSAC,CND	1 CUP	10	260
SPAGHETTI,MEATBALLS,TOMSA,HMRP	1 CUP	12	330
SPECIAL K CEREAL	1 OZ	0	110
SPINACH SOUFFLE	1 CUP	18	220
SPINACH, CANNED, DRND,W/ SALT	1 CUP	1	50
SPINACH, CANNED, DRND,W/O SALT	1 CUP	1	50
SPINACH, COOKED FR FRZEN, DRND	1 CUP	0	55
SPINACH, COOKED FROM RAW, DRND	1 CUP	0	40
SPINACH, RAW	1 CUP	0	10
SQUASH, SUMMER, COOKED, DRAIN	1 CUP	1	35
SQUASH, WINTER, BAKED	1 CUP	1	80
STRAWBERRIES, FROZEN, SWEETEN	1 CUP	0	245
STRAWBERRIES, FROZEN, SWEETEN	10 OZ	0	275
STRAWBERRIES, RAW	1 CUP	1	45
SUGAR COOKIE, FROM REFRIG DOGH	4 COOKIE	12	235
SUGAR FROSTED FLAKES, KELLOGG	1 OZ	0	110
SUGAR SMACKS CEREAL	1 OZ	1	105
SUGAR, BROWN, PRESSED DOWN	1 CUP	0	820
SUGAR, POWDERED, SIFTED	1 CUP	0	385
SUGAR, WHITE, GRANULATED	1 CUP	0	770
SUGAR, WHITE, GRANULATED	1 PKT	0	25
SUGAR, WHITE, GRANULATED	1 TBSP	0	45
SUNFLOWER OIL	1 CUP	218	1925
SUNFLOWER OIL	1 TBSP	14	125
SUNFLOWER SEEDS	1 OZ	14	160
SUPER SUGAR CRISP CEREAL	1 OZ	0	105
SWEET (DARK) CHOCOLATE	1 OZ	10	150
SWEETENED CONDENSED MILK CNND	1 CUP	27	980
SWEETPOTATOES, BAKED, PEELED	1 POTATO	0	115
SWEETPOTATOES, BOILED W/O PEEL	1 POTATO	0	160
SWEETPOTATOES, CANDIED	1 PIECE	3	145
SWEETPOTATOES, CANNED, MASHED	1 CUP	1	260

Description of food		Fat (grams)	Food Energy (calories)
SWEETPOTATOES, CNNED, VAC PACK	1 PIECE	0	35
SWISS CHEESE	1 OZ	8	105
SYRUP, CHOCOLATE FLAVORED THIN	2 TBSP	0	85
SYRUP, CHOCOLATE FLVRED, FUDGE	2 TBSP	5	125
TABLE SYRUP (CORN AND MAPLE)	2 TBSP	0	122
TACO	1 TACO	11	195
TAHINI	1 TBSP	8	90
TANGERINE JUICE, CANNED, SWTNED	1 CUP	0	125
TANGERINES, CANNED, LIGHT SYRP	1 CUP	0	155
TANGERINES, RAW	1 TANGRN	0	35
TARTAR SAUCE	1 TBSP	8	75
TEA, BREWED	8 FL OZ	0	0
TEA, INSTANT, PREPRD, UNSWEETEN	D8 FL OZ	0	0
TEA, INSTANT, PREPARD, SWEETENED	8 FL OZ	0	85
TOASTER PASTRIES	1 PASTRY	6	210
TOFU	1 PIECE	5	85
TOMATO JUICE, CANNED WITH SALT	1 CUP	0	40
TOMATO JUICE, CANNED W/O SALT	1 CUP	0	40
TOMATO PASTE, CANNED WITH SALT	1 CUP	2	220
TOMATO PASTE, CANNED W/O SALT	1 CUP	2	220
TOMATO PUREE, CANNED WITH SALT	1 CUP	0	105
TOMATO PUREE, CANNED W/O SALT	1 CUP	0	105
TOMATO SAUCE, CANNED WITH SALT	1 CUP	0	75
TOMATO SOUP WITH MILK, CANNED	1 CUP	6	160
TOMATO SOUP W/ WATER, CANNED	1 CUP	2	85
TOMATO VEG SOUP, DEHYD, PREPRED	1 PKT	1	40
TOMATOES, CANNED, S+L, W/ SALT	1 CUP	1	50
TOMATOES, CANNED, S+L, W/O SALT	1 CUP	1	50
TOMATOES, RAW	1 TOMATO	0	25
TORTILLAS, CORN	1 TORTLA	1	65
TOTAL CEREAL	1 OZ	1	100
TRIX CEREAL	1 OZ	0	110
TROUT, BROILED, W/ BUTTR, LEMJU	3 OZ	9	175
TUNA SALAD	1 CUP	19	375
TUNA, CANND, DRND, OIL, CHK, LGHT	3 OZ	7	165
TUNA, CANND, DRND, WATR, WHITE	3 OZ	1	135
TURKEY HAM, CURED TURKEY THIGH	2 SLICES	3	75

Description of food		Fat (grams)	Food Energy (calories)
TURKEY LOAF, BREAST MEAT W/O C2	SLICES	1	45
TURKEY LOAF, BREAST MEAT, W/ C2	SLICES	1	45
TURKEY PATTIES, BRD,BATTD,FRID1	PATTY	12	180
TURKEY ROAST, FRZN,LGHT+DRK,CK3	OZ	5	130
TURKEY, ROASTED, DARK MEAT 4	PIECES	6	160
TURKEY, ROASTED, LIGHT MEAT 2	PIECES	3	135
TURKEY, ROASTED, LIGHT + DARK 1	CUP	7	240
TURKEY, ROASTED, LIGHT + DARK 3	PIECES	4	145
TURNIP GREENS, CKED FRM FROZEN1	CUP	1	50
TURNIP GREENS, COOKED FROM RAW1	CUP	0	30
TURNIPS, COOKED, DICED 1	CUP	0	30
VANILLA WAFERS 10	COOKE	7	185
VEAL CUTLET, MED FAT,BRSD,BRLD3	OZ	9	185
VEAL RIB, MED FAT, ROASTED 3	OZ	14	230
VEGETABLE BEEF SOUP, CANNED 1	CUP	2	80
VEGETABLE JUICE COCKTAIL, CNND1	CUP	0	45
VEGETABLES, MIXED, CANNED 1	CUP	0	75
VEGETABLES, MIXED, CKED FR FRZ1	CUP	0	105
VEGETARIAN SOUP, CANNED 1	CUP	2	70
VIENNA BREAD 1	SLICE	1	70
VIENNA SAUSAGE 1	SAUSAG	4	45
VINEGAR AND OIL SALAD DRESSING1	TBSP	8	70
VINEGAR, CIDER 1	TBSP	0	0
WAFFLES, FROM HOME RECIPE 1	WAFFLE	13	245
WAFFLES, FROM MIX 1	WAFFLE	8	205
WALNUTS, BLACK, CHOPPED 1	CUP	71	760
WALNUTS, BLACK, CHOPPED 1	OZ	16	170
WALNUTS, ENGLISH, PIECES 1	CUP	74	770
WALNUTS, ENGLISH, PIECES 1	OZ	18	180
WATER CHESTNUTS, CANNED 1	CUP	0	70
WATERMELON, RAW 1	PIECE	2	155
WATERMELON, RAW, DICED 1	CUP	1	50
WHEAT BREAD 1	LOAF	19	1160
WHEAT BREAD 1	SLICE	1	65
WHEAT BREAD, TOASTED 1	SLICE	1	65
WHEAT FLOUR, ALL-PURPOSE,SIFTD1	CUP	1	420
WHEAT FLOUR, ALL-PURPOSE,UNSIF1	CUP	1	455

Description of food		Fat (grams)	Food Energy (calories)
WHEATIES CEREAL	1 OZ	0	100
WHEAT, THIN CRACKERS	4 CRACKR	1	35
WHIPPED TOPPING, PRESSURIZED	1 CUP	13	155
WHIPPED TOPPING, PRESSURIZED	1 TBSP	1	10
WHIPPING CREAM, UNWHIPED,HEAVY	1 CUP	88	820
WHIPPING CREAM, UNWHIPED,HEAVY	1 TBSP	6	50
WHIPPING CREAM, UNWHIPED,LIGHT	1 CUP	74	700
WHIPPING CREAM, UNWHIPED,LIGHT	1 TBSP	5	45
WHITE BREAD	1 LOAF	18	1210
WHITE BREAD CRUMBS, SOFT	1 CUP	2	120
WHITE BREAD CUBES	1 CUP	1	80
WHITE BREAD, SLICE 18 PER LOAF	1 SLICE	1	65
WHITE BREAD, SLICE 22 PER LOAF	1 SLICE	1	55
WHITE BREAD, TOASTED 18 PER	1 SLICE	1	65
WHITE BREAD, TOASTED 22 PER	1 SLICE	1	55
WHITE CAKE W/ WHT FRSTNG,COMML	1 CAKE	148	4170
WHITE CAKE W/ WHT FRSTNG,COMML	1 PIECE	9	260
WHITE SAUCE W/ MILK FROM MIX	1 CUP	13	240
WHITE SAUCE, MEDIUM, HOME RECP	1 CUP	30	395
WHOLE-WHEAT BREAD	1 LOAF	20	1110
WHOLE-WHEAT BREAD	1 SLICE	1	70
WHOLE-WHEAT BREAD, TOASTED	1 SLICE	1	70
WHOLE-WHEAT FLOUR,HRD WHT,STIR	1 CUP	2	400
WHOLE-WHEAT WAFERS, CRACKERS	2 CRACKR	2	35
WINE, DESSERT	3.5 F OZ	0	140
WINE, TABLE, RED	3.5 F OZ	0	75
WINE, TABLE, WHITE	3.5 F OZ	0	80
YEAST, BAKERS, DRY, ACTIVE	1 PKG	0	20
YEAST, BREWERS, DRY	1 TBSP	0	25
YELLOW CAKE W/ CHOC FRST,FRMIX	1 CAKE	125	3735
YELLOW CAKE W/ CHOC FRST,FRMIX	1 PIECE	8	235
YELLOWCAKE W/ CHOCFRSTNG,COMML	1 CAKE	175	3895
YELLOWCAKE W/ CHOCFRSTNG,COMML	1 PIECE	11	245
YOGURT, W/ LOFAT MILK, PLAIN	8 OZ	4	145
YOGURT, W/ LOFAT MILK,FRUITFLV	8 OZ	2	230
YOGURT, W/ NONFAT MILK	8 OZ	0	125
YOGURT, W/ WHOLE MILK	8 OZ	7	140